WHY
DOULAS
MATTER

Pinter & Martin Why it Matters

There is more **information** *available on giving birth and raising children* **than** *ever before. With each new scientific advance or fad,* **more** *questions arise. The Why It Matters series seeks to steer* **a** *course through this sea of information, and offer* **succinct**, *balanced and evidence-based introductions to* **a wide** *range of subjects, giving readers a firm framework* **from** *which to make confident, informed decisions of their own.*

Spring 2015

1 Why the Politics of Breastfeeding Matter
2 Why Hypnobirthing Matters
3 Why Doulas Matter

Autumn 2015

4 Why Pre-Conception and Pregnancy Nutrition Matters
5 Why Breastfeeding Matters
6 Why Baby-Led Weaning Matters

2016 and beyond

Why Your Baby's Sleep Matters | Why Perinatal Depression Matters | Why Babywearing Matters | Why Your Birth Experience Matters | Why VBAC Matters | Why Attachment Parenting Matters | Why Home Birth Matters | Why Midwives Matter | Why Fathers Matter | Why Tests in Pregnancy Matter *and many more*

for the latest titles, please visit
pinterandmartin.com/why-it-matters

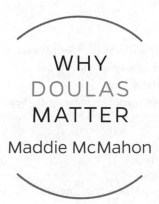

WHY
DOULAS
MATTER

Maddie McMahon

pinter
&
martin

Why Doulas Matter (Pinter & Martin Why It Matters: 3)

First published by Pinter & Martin Ltd 2015

© 2015 Maddie McMahon

Maddie McMahon has asserted her moral right to be identified as the author of this work in accordance with the Copyright, Designs and Patents Act of 1988.

All rights reserved

ISBN 978-1-78066-510-8
Also available as ebook

Pinter & Martin Why It Matters ISSN 2056-8657

Series editor: Susan Last
Index: Helen Bilton
Proofreader: Debbie Kennett

British Library Cataloguing-in-Publication Data
A catalogue record for this book is available from the British Library.

Set in Minion

Printed and bound in the UK by Ashford Colour Press Ltd, Gosport, Hampshire

This book has been printed on paper that is sourced and harvested from sustainable forests and is FSC accredited.

Pinter & Martin Ltd
6 Effra Parade
London SW2 1PS

pinterandmartin.com

Contents

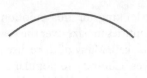

Introduction

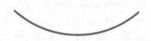

*Doula: A woman who gives support, help, and advice
to another woman during pregnancy and during and
after the birth.*

Oxford English Dictionary

It's 5.30am. Weak rays of sun are beginning to illuminate the hospital multi-storey car park. I sit in the driver's seat and pause a minute, yawning, before turning the key in the ignition.

I smell. My teeth are furry. My back, legs and feet ache like I've just run a marathon. I've eaten nothing but a panini from the coffee shop, a banana and glucose tablets for 36 hours and I'm hungry. And oh, so tired. I pull my rebozo tighter around my cold shoulders and smile. I am exalting; brimming over with admiration and pride. My soul is still sitting with the woman I have just accompanied through her journey to motherhood. The look of pure joy on her face as her child emerged into the water and the waiting hands of her husband is still engraved on my heart.

I never went looking for this emotional rollercoaster. I tried on many identities for size over the years before giving in and answering the call. Many of us realise that we have been doulas all our lives. Contrary to popular assumption, doulas have always been here. We kept the wolf from the door when we birthed in caves; we probably came to that famous stable.

We have many names and none. We are that woman in the village who always knows when your time is close. We appear with food, love, warm water and strong arms. We shepherd the children, call the midwife and hold the mother as she and her baby work together towards birth. We are witch, godmother, wisewoman, sister. The antecedent of the midwife; some of us learnt which herbs stop bleeding and how to help if a baby is stuck, or malpositioned. Some of us still journey on to midwifery. And some midwives end up as doulas.

As Adela Stockton, author of *Gentle Birth Companions*, the definitive text on the UK and European doula movement attests:

> *While a doula…may aspire to improve the standard of her knowledge, the real essence of the doula comes from within herself and is not necessarily something that can be taught.*

It is in this fundamental way that we differ from midwives, who bear the clinical responsibility for the wellbeing of mother and baby, as well as traditionally providing psycho-social support. Midwifery training has a large emphasis on academic attainment. Doula preparation is almost entirely about self-knowledge, self-development, and the practice of social and emotional intelligence.

The title of this book is a statement that I have been grappling with for over a decade. On one level, doulas do not matter. It is all about the parents. Their journey, their feelings, their experience of childbirth and early parenting. To serve, to me, means to provide succour and to minister to the every need of my clients as they negotiate an intense period in their lives. My needs are secondary. Ego plays no part. How I feel and what I think, my memories and my opinions, have no place in their story.

Yet here I am, charged with trying to describe what doulas do, to give you a glimpse into our strange and rather obsessive world and to explain why I think we do make a difference. I want to give free rein to the voices of the parents and doulas who populate my world.

Doulas are just women who really, truly care about other women, on a major level.

Linda Quinn, doula and doula mentor

The realisation that a woman, experienced in childbirth, who is neither a member of the hospital staff, nor a part of the mother's social circle, can have a tangible, positive effect on both the woman's experience of childbirth and the outcomes of that labour, first began to dawn in the 1970s and 80s. Following on from their famous work on mother-infant bonding, paediatricians Klaus and Kennell's studies of doula-support led to the founding of Doulas of North America (DONA) in the early 1990s. The research has continued, most recently with a Cochrane review that found such beneficial effects of doula support that it recommended all woman have access to it.

In the UK, well-known obstetrician Michel Odent was instrumental in the founding of Doula UK in 2001. It has built a community of support, ongoing learning and mentoring. At first, it was a coming together of women who, more often than not, were doulas and didn't know it. They were asked to accompany a mother through childbirth and the early days with the baby and found they had a natural aptitude for the role. There was no 'training' as such. What evolved as our organisation grew was a new need for some preparation for the role and then, once the woman had started supporting mothers and fathers, opportunities for mentoring and reflection.

Doula courses began to appear. These encourage a woman to reflect on her own story, what being a doula means to her, and crucially, the boundaries of the role. Courses are not academic 'training' – course leaders seek to empower, inform and nurture the woman, encouraging her to access her emotional intelligence and empathic powers. It is only by receiving these things, that we can hope to pass them on. We need to 'be doulaed' in order to doula others.

This word 'support' is one we use a lot. It is both a noun and verb, used to mean to hold up, help, approve of, to take care of and provide for, to advocate and defend. These definitions certainly go some way to explaining what doulas do.

A 'three-legged stool' underpins our work: practical, emotional and informational support. Practically, we cook, we clean, we accompany on hospital visits, we entertain children, we hold her up through contractions, massage her, remind her partner to eat and sleep and show him how he can support her. We change nappies, teach parents how to wear their babies, walk miles pushing prams while mothers sleep, sit with her while she and her baby perfect the dance that is breastfeeding. We mop brows and make the tea.

As we drink the tea, we listen:

> *[Her] understanding and kindness really helped me work through [my fears] and by the time my due date was near, I was actually looking forward to everything starting! ...I felt safe and looked after.*

Providing information or pointing parents to sources of knowledge and support is the last leg of the stool. This 'signposting' can include providing contacts for services such as antenatal education, complementary therapies or midwifery or obstetric support. We might support our clients through the process of informed decision-making, pointing them towards websites, books or research that may provide the missing pieces of the puzzle.

> *[She] listened to our concerns, provided crucial information, care and understanding in a completely non-judgemental, non-prescriptive way. She opened our minds to options and choices that were available to us and encouraged me to trust in my instincts and feelings about the birth I wanted.*

I often stumble on internet forums where women are discussing doulas. They ask many questions, make assumptions and perpetuate myths. But really, all anyone needs to know about doulas is that the relationship with her will be unique. Doulas can be found in hospitals, in birth centres and at home; in large houses, small flats, boats, tents, prisons and even in the birth pool. We are sometimes a woman's sole support and often part of a circle around the mother.

A doula is 'the woman who serves': ask a doula what you need and she will give. A doula is a woman who offers: she will bring forgotten ritual, ceremony and community back into your life, fulfilling a yearning you may never know you had.

A doula should have no agenda and no judgement. She looks in the mirror daily and repeats the mantra, 'it's not about me'. Her passion is to walk the path with you, supporting you unconditionally. Put simply, her role is to nurture – through her love and care, mothers can focus their energies on loving and caring for their babies.

I am often asked how we get on with maternity services. I

spent years being ignored in birth rooms, being assumed to be the sister (and latterly, due to the grey hair, the grandma). I have smiled and tried to be kind and accommodating. I have made many marvellous midwife friends. These days, in part due to the overwhelming evidence that doulas have a positive effect on birth outcomes, the NHS and other organisations are becoming more open to working with us. There are schemes around the country working hard to offer support to women in need. There are even some schemes where the doula is provided by the hospital, when you are in labour. For me, the magic of the doula is about the mother doing the choosing, so ideally no doula should ever be 'assigned' to a mother without her having the final say.

If you are a mother, father, midwife, doula or doctor reading this book, you may recognise feelings described within these pages. If you don't relate to any of it, I'm sorry. If I've learned one thing as a doula, it's that everyone's experience is uniquely theirs. When it comes to pregnancy, childbirth and babycare, it can be hard to find common ground. It can be tough not to judge or to feel judged in turn. It is important for me to say to you, dear reader, what I say to my clients: I have no agenda, other than offering you options and information and supporting you to find the way that suits you best.

This book is not intended to tell you what is right or wrong, give you advice or tell you what to do. The thoughts and experiences in this book come from my years working with parents and learning what appears to support them through the transition to parenthood. I try my best to be guided by the best available evidence but, in the end, anyone who thinks they know what is best for you is being ridiculous: only a mother is the expert on her own body and her own baby.

NB: In the interests of easy reading, partners are male and babies are female in this book. I know it can be the other way round too!

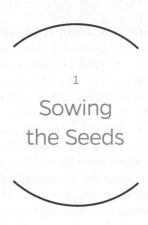

1

Sowing the Seeds

Sally knew she wanted me as her doula. I had supported her after having her first child and we had become friends. Having her first baby had been very hard on her, physically and emotionally, and so it had taken her a long time and lots of talking to feel ready to have another baby.

I felt a little guilty when I heard that I was the first person she'd told about the 'blue line'; not even her husband knew yet. 'Will you be my doula?' she asked, with a tremor in her voice. I knew she was scared. 'I already am', I told her. 'Now, put the phone down and ring Peter.'

Sally's body and mind were as ready as they could be for this pregnancy. But she had needed to heal from the mental scars left by a frightening first birth. It had taken quite some time for her to be ready to lie on her sofa and allow me to invite her to go back, in her imagination, to that first birth experience. She told me about the shouting, the coercion and how overwhelmed she felt when she was told she needed to go to theatre for a forceps delivery. While all around her were celebrating the birth of a healthy child, she felt cold, numb and struggled to feed and bond with her baby.

This time, she was determined, things would be different. And they were. Her son was born in water, at home, into the gentle hands of his father, watched by her midwife and me. She was surrounded by love and admiration.

Many of us, especially first time, walk into pregnancy with our eyes firmly shut. Other than possibly taking a prenatal vitamin supplement, we know little of how we might prepare our bodies or our minds for the conception of a child. The immense transformation that growing and birthing a person has on the psyche needs, I believe, physical and emotional support so that we don't come out of the other side of the experience depleted at some elemental level.

Women come to pregnancy in all manner of ways. There is no right or wrong, just what life gives us. I have known women who have conceived in violence and fear, others in love. Some with intent and others by accident. Most come to love and want their babies, while others take the decision to terminate. Sometimes, nature decides for them and the child is lost. My role, whatever the circumstances, is to love and support that woman.

People often ask me when the best time is to begin a relationship with a doula. My answer is always, 'when you feel the need of some support'. Early pregnancy can be a particularly hard time, sometimes made more difficult by a culture that imposes a vow of secrecy on parents for at least the first trimester. I have often wondered why it is that, at a time when a woman can be feeling dog-tired, nauseous, scared and emotionally overwhelmed, she has very few people to turn to, other than her partner, for support. Her partner may be feeling rather wobbly himself: pregnancy can seem unreal and worries about money and the responsibilities of parenthood can cause a lot of stress.

Not all conceptions make it the full nine months, so if a woman loses a baby in the first trimester, she has to explain her grief to people who didn't even know she was pregnant. A miscarriage is not an embarrassment or a shame to be hidden. Telling people is certainly not tempting fate and risking the worst happening. But if you're superstitious or enjoying keeping the secret, you can of course hug that wonderful knowledge to yourself for a while and enjoy it.

Both before conception and during the early weeks of pregnancy, a doula can be a useful additional support. Whether you intend to grow your baby, birth her and keep her or not, having someone to listen to your feelings, offering a shoulder, useful suggestions and introductions to people who may be able to help you can be extremely comforting. A doula makes no moral judgements and will go to the grave with your secrets.

One of my favourite doulas works a lot in the realm of pre-conception. She is often approached by women who are struggling to conceive. What Suzanne gives, that is often so difficult to find in the IVF clinics and hospital waiting rooms, is a warm, loving faith in the woman's body and an understanding that our minds can affect the body's abilities. I know women who feel that just meeting Suzanne shifted a mental block or brought a deeply hidden anxiety to the surface. Perhaps her warm hands on their feet during a reflexology session decrease stress hormones and allow the hormones of love and conception to flow freely. Whatever is happening, since becoming a doula I have learned over and over that women need more than just white coats, drugs and cold, hard science to conceive, grow and birth a child.

I feel that we have a deep primal instinct that knows at a physical/biological level at times of stress/anxiety [that] it's not good to bring a new baby into our world. Our womanly instinct protects both mother and child. In today's fast-paced world it can sometimes be a challenge to conceive and the emotional pain of infertility can create even more stress hormones. I have found that through trust and faith in our amazing female bodies, it's possible with love and support to release stress and create a positive mind set, becoming aligned with conception in mind, body and soul.

Suzanne Howlett

Tilda had lost her husband a few years before. He died tragically and with no warning, just as they were beginning to try to conceive a child. Along with the grief of not having a child, comes the grief that it will never be *his* child. But there came a time, after years of wondering if she'd meet someone else, that she decided that emotionally and financially, she was at the right point in her life to become a mother.

Maria, a novelist, bought sperm on the internet and told me the story of meeting her donor, his face covered with a motorcycle helmet, at a service station, to swap cash for a small vial filled with hope.

In this way a doula may be involved from the start, to the extent of being present at the conception. The very medical nature of most assisted conceptions can be an emotional rollercoaster. To support her own body's powers and to bring a personal touch to her conception, Tilda searched for things she could do to help the treatment succeed. After talking things through with her doula, she used acupuncture to enhance her fertility. There is some research that supports the use of acupuncture during IVF treatment, but for me the psychological advantage of giving the parents a little bit of calm and control is equally important.

Single women and same-sex couples not only have to

endure the indignity of assisted conception and all the physical challenges that entails, but also sometimes have to deal with the judgement and confusion of a society that is still not quite used to the idea that there are many types of family. Once you are pregnant, people tend to ask difficult questions, forget to include your same-sex partner in discussions and decisions, or worry about your ability to cope as a single parent.

I have grown so used to these once-unusual scenarios that it doesn't even occur to me to ask how the baby was conceived. None of it seems outlandish to me; every one of those women is just a mother who needs my support.

You might have been hoping and dreaming for a baby for a long time, got pregnant very quickly, or be coming to terms with an accidental conception. If you are aiming to keep your baby, what now? These days, pregnancy tests are so good that some women know they are pregnant even before they are due to have their period. It could be some weeks before you meet a midwife for the first time for your 'booking in' appointment. It is at this meeting that the scene is often set for the rest of the pregnancy. If women are treated kindly, don't feel like they are being rushed, or judged or interrogated, the foundation of trust in their caregivers is created. I often hear great stories about first appointments, but sometimes women tell me it was a 'blood-letting and tick-box exercise', with no real attempt to get to know them or provide emotional support.

If you are a woman living in an area where it is unlikely that you'll ever meet the same midwife again, it's hardly surprising she made no attempt to bond with you. This is not only a sad state of affairs for you – continuity of care has been proven time and again to be safer for you and the baby – but also for the midwives, who no longer have the satisfaction of building relationships with mothers and their families.

Once you begin to find out what maternity care looks like

in your area, you may begin to think about what you want and need in this pregnancy. I am always a little sad when parents come to me seeking doula support because they have realised they will not have the opportunity to get to know a midwife. I have no ambition to replace the holistic, nurturing, therapeutic relationship a woman should have with her midwife – a midwife who should ideally care for her before, during and after the birth of her baby. It is natural for our species to need the support of other women during the transition to motherhood. Like elephants, dolphins and bonobos, we seek the safety of female companions. When those relationships are absent, we seek them out. Doula? Midwife? It's not an either-or. A doula should complement your relationship with your midwife. A pregnant woman can't have too much love and care.

Why be 'doulaed'?

Women seek out doula support for a whole host of reasons. Sometimes it is the partners who reach out first and need us more than the mothers. There is no normal – just you and your story. Here are just some of the reasons parents have sought me out.

Birth doula support

- They are anxious first-timers who want some support from an experienced mother.
- They want a 'teacher' – someone to tell them what to do.
- They are immigrants or visitors to the UK who feel they need a guide through an alien maternity system.
- They are new to the area and therefore have no friends and family on hand.
- She's a single mother with no other source of practical support.
- They are dealing with trauma from a previous experience.
- They are hoping for a natural birth of twins or planning

a vaginal birth after caesarean (VBAC).
- They need an extra pair of hands at a homebirth to help care for older children.
- He is terrified so needs someone to keep him calm and allow him to come and go during the birth.
- They have realised they will have no continuity of care and want a consistent friendly face.
- Because religious beliefs or cultural practices mean the man is not in the birth room.
- Because they crave a mother/sister figure who is missing in their lives.
- Because they've had a doula before and they loved it.
- Because a friend or midwife or obstetrician suggests they get a doula.
- Because they have no idea how to arrange the birth they want.
- Because it just feels right to have a female birth companion.
- Because a friend or relative had a doula and said it was marvellous!
- Because the parents have experienced the loss of a baby and this time they need lots of extra love.

Postnatal doula support
- Life is overwhelming and tiring and she just needs to sleep and talk about how she feels.
- She needs help with a toddler or school age child while she 'babymoons'.
- She could do with some practical help around the house because she had a caesarean.
- Caring for a newborn is alien territory – they want a 'teacher'.
- Multiples – all hands on deck!

- She is suffering from postnatal depression and the family needs extra support.
- She suffered from PND last time and wants to avoid it this time!
- She is a single mother with no family support.
- She is worried about bonding or breastfeeding.
- Because postnatal support is usual in their country! (Dutch parents, for example, get daily practical support in the home provided by the state).
- Because they crave a mother/sister figure who is missing in their lives.
- Because one or both of the children have special needs
- Because the parents have special needs, learning difficulties or mental health issues.
- Because if the mother doesn't get just one full night of sleep, she doesn't know what she'll do (night-doulaing).
- Because other stressful issues are happening simultaneously – bereavements or financial crises for example.
- Because she is finding the transition to motherhood is challenging her sense of identity.
- Because they had a doula last time and she was such a great help.
- Because they are super-anxious about caring for a new baby.

Choosing a doula

Just as there are myriad reasons for working with a doula, there is endless variation in the doula-client relationship. The path may have many twists and turns. The journey may be long or challenging in any number of ways. Travelling companions need to, at the very least, trust each other and, ideally, like each other. In fact I have found that we all feel the best in the end if I've found something, anything, I can genuinely love in my clients.

Choosing a doula may be difficult or easy. You may have lots of choice or very little. This will depend on geography – how many doulas are within a reasonable distance of you – and other factors, like how quickly the local doulas get booked up, whether it's a busy time of year (April and September are my busiest months – summer and Christmas conceptions!) and how many clients your local doulas are taking on. It makes sense to start looking around and putting out some feelers as soon as you begin to think that you might want a doula. It will be useful to reflect on when you might want the most support: during pregnancy and labour, or after the baby is born? Or both? This will help you work out whether you need a birth doula, a postnatal doula or both. Many of us offer both birth and postnatal support, but you may find you need two doulas to create your dream team.

Thinking about the kind of person you feel comfortable inviting into your space is important. One client admitted that she took me on because I wore clothes that suggested I had no hippy tendencies. She laughingly told me that she quickly realised how wrong about me she had been, but that she had learned how unimportant any of that stuff is.

> *I knew what I wanted from a doula and knew that... despite being her first client, she would be everything I needed. [Even though] I wouldn't choose to have my family with me while I labour... I chose [my doula] because she reminded me of my sister. I got the comfort and security I needed while being away from family. After an informal chat I asked her back to meet my husband to make sure he felt comfortable with her too.*
>
> Kristal Rees

You may be the kind of person who likes structure and

guidance in situations like this. After all, many of us have never employed anyone's services before meeting a doula. You might like the list of questions to ask a birth or postnatal doula on the Doula UK website. But you might find that the chat just flows. I never feel comfortable with being the *talker* at a first meeting. This whole thing after all is about *the parents*. Like most shy people I'd much prefer to be asking you some nice open questions and listening. I am genuinely interested in your story, why you want a doula, whether both parents are on the same page and what your differing needs may be.

Being open and up front about the financial side of things is crucial. If you're financially unable to afford to pay a fee for your doula, tell her – she will have lots of ideas up her sleeve. The Doula UK Access Fund, vouchers for friends and family to buy you as gifts, bartering and payment in kind are just some of the ways we doulas manage to support our communities.

I'm sometimes asked if it's upsetting when a couple meets with a few doulas and I'm not the one who is picked. I can honestly say no. I've learned over the years that if I am not drawn to a couple or I'm not floating their boat, then working together would be no fun anyway. It might even end up feeling negative for both parties. The only thing I care about is that the parents find the right doula for them.

I once knocked on a front door at around 8pm on a blustery winter night. I was on a mercy mission, answering a call from a stressed father about his wife, who was crying in pain every time her baby nursed. He answered the door immediately and ushered me in. There was no sign of a pram in the hall, nor could I see or hear any other evidence that there was a woman or baby in the house. As he closed the door behind me, icy fingers squeezed my heart. Thankfully, he disappeared briefly upstairs and his wife soon appeared on the landing, gesturing me to come up.

So if you're a dad and you call a doula, she will ask to speak to your partner before she comes to your house. She'll really appreciate it if you tell her where she can safely park and anything else useful about your neighbourhood that will help her find you safely. And if she's with you more than a couple of hours, don't be surprised if her phone beeps; there may well be someone anxiously awaiting her at home.

Definitions

Defining a doula is a tricky task. Although we were very excited to make it into the *Oxford English Dictionary* a few years back, the real definition is more fluid. A doula will probably be a 'lay woman' – not a health professional – and she won't be offering clinical care. She may be part of your community or live some distance away. She may charge for her services, or just ask for her expenses to be covered. She might want paying with money or be happy with a skills swap or payment in kind. She may come to you via another agency or you may seek her out yourself. You might meet a doula because you are pregnant in prison, or because you need more social support through a tough time in your life. She might be a volunteer for an organisation or run her own business.

A doula may be young, old or anywhere in between. We come in all colours of the rainbow, all religious persuasions and sexual orientations. She might even, perhaps, be a man – but that is another discussion! She may or may not be a mother herself. She might offer you additional services alongside doula support. She may be straight and scientific, business-like, informal, hippy or spiritual: or anything else. There is no pinning down the definition of a doula.

There truly is a 'doula for every woman' – the important thing is that you choose one with your heart as well as your head.

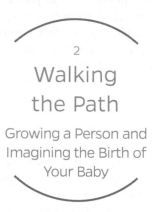

2
Walking
the Path
Growing a Person and
Imagining the Birth of
Your Baby

I must irritate my clients sometimes: they want answers and they are hard to provide. They ask 'piece of string' questions like 'When will I have my baby?' 'How long will labour be?' and 'Will it hurt?' My answer is often, 'Nobody knows'. Other questions, like 'When should I go to hospital?' or 'How do I know when my baby is hungry?' can only be answered with 'You will know'.

As a culture, we often neglect to explain that, while parenting is instinctive, those instincts can be easily interrupted. High-tech birth interventions, parenting 'gurus' and social attitudes that encourage the separation of mother and baby all distance us from our mammalian instincts. Parents are told to ignore what their hearts are telling them and follow the prescribed rules set down by hospitals, doctors, authors and other parents. These 'rules' may have some benefit to a population as a whole, while others are arbitrary nonsense with no logic or scientific evidence behind them, and some are cultural norms or traditions. Not all will benefit *you* as an individual.

Rules, pathways, policies and protocols can't take into account your personal preferences or feelings.

In this climate we have forgotten something: women know a lot about their bodies and their babies. They have information no doctor can access. During labour, if it's sore and you move to ease that sensation, you will be working with your baby to guide her towards the exit. When you just 'know' your baby needs to be born by caesarean, despite what the doctors say, there will be a reason that is as valid as any medical explanation. If your baby cries and your heart yearns to pick her up, you will be giving her the psychological nurturing she needs to grow into a healthy, balanced child and adult. If your breasts feel full and you want to nurse, I bet she fancies a snack or needs the comfort of your warm skin and sweet smell.

We carry our whole selves into parenthood: the way we were born and brought up, and all our experiences and learning inform our journey and influence the decisions we make along the way. This is our 'internal birth dialogue': conversations we have with ourselves about what birth is like. Some of us grew up with mothers who birthed and nursed their children with ease. Increasingly, however, our Western culture has separated us from this deep trust in the process. Birth has become a scary, dangerous enterprise from which we must be rescued by experts. Baby care has morphed into something that needs to be dictated, rather than explored and enjoyed in response to our babies' cues.

When you recognise how you have defined childbirth, and where it is filed in your mind, you can begin to explore where those assumptions and ideas have come from and perhaps deconstruct them and replace them with something more realistic, more positive and more useful.

Getting to know you during pregnancy will also help your

doula support you during labour. As we chat over a cup of tea we begin to find out who you are and what you might need. This process can have ripple effects on the whole family for years to come:

> *When you visited me at home antenatally, you asked me what I do when I feel overwhelmed or stressed and I said that I go hide. You asked what I want in this situation. And I replied 'I want to be followed, obviously!'… When I went and hid in the toilet in transition, my husband didn't come to find me, but you remembered and you did. Reflecting on this moment and others actually helps me communicate with my husband better – I need to let him know in times of calm what helps me in moments of stress.*
> Abigail Salehi

Making friends with your body

We live in a society that views the female body in a rather confused and contradictory manner. Our bodies are meant to be attractive and function perfectly. We are praised if we expose our bodies to the approving gaze of others, but conversely called all sorts of names if we expose too much, or at an inappropriate moment. The 'rules' of this game are complicated: cleavage is good (unless it's a job interview); areola and nipple is bad. Hair on head is good, anywhere else it's dirty and offensive. Menstrual blood is gross and must be hidden, along with the emotional ebbs and flows that go with it. We are taught to buff and primp and show off our bodies, yet hide ourselves away and take the blame and shame if we expose too much.

Living in a society in which bodies are displayed for others' consumption and entertainment does a number of things to a woman. I've met women who have decided to spend a lot of time on the body-beautiful. At the other end of the spectrum are those who have chosen to ignore their bodies, who have upped sticks and moved to live, almost entirely, in their heads.

Both these states can have an impact on the way women approach childbirth. Your body is going to change and rearrange itself in ways you never thought possible. And it's going to *make* you notice. You can choose whether to be repelled or to feel proud of your body's magical properties. You can create a new person. Whether you need someone's help to birth your baby or whether you do it all by yourself, the fact remains, you *made* a *person*. That is an amazing thing.

As leading American midwife Ina May Gaskin so memorably says:

> *There is no other organ quite like the uterus. If men had such an organ they would brag about it. So should we.*

It makes me sad when women are afraid of their bodies, or disgusted by them, or fear they will break down, not be up to the challenge or be spoilt by childbirth, leaving them fat, saggy and unattractive. Actually, many fathers I work with tell me they've never seen their partners looking so beautiful. They are in awe. And your baby? Well, your body is her home, her why and wherefore, her everything. When you see your body through the eyes of those who love you – your baby and partner – how does it feel?

I've found that it can pay huge dividends if we 'make friends with our bodies' before and during pregnancy. Now is the time to get to know how you work and build pride and confidence in your body's abilities. I might be about to sound like a 1970s hippy-feminist, but how well do you know your vagina? Can you name all the parts? Are you aware of its amazing capabilities? Some of my clients have found it incredibly confidence-boosting to do perineal massage. I don't think we necessarily *need* to do this in order to let out a baby without tearing – nature has come up with a spongy, stretchy vagina that usually does a pretty good job. But spending some time becoming familiar with that area, experiencing the sensation of stretching and not being afraid to touch yourself can pay off when you are pushing your baby out.

Fear can be lessened and pleasure zones can be utilised to allow you to stretch and open more efficiently. It can be overwhelmingly wonderful to put your finger inside yourself when you are pushing and feel the top of your baby's head.

The parts of your body through which your baby will pass are the same as those that allowed you to conceive and give you sexual pleasure. In fact, the basic ingredients for good love-making and orgasm are the same as for labour and birth. The environment and the hormones are exactly the same – and crucially, for both birth and orgasm to 'work', a shutting down of the inhibition centres of the brain is vital.

Did you know your breasts are already getting themselves ready to be your baby's 'womb in the world'? They are growing more milk-making equipment and even beginning to make colostrum – the baby's first milk. Once your baby is born, your breasts are nature's incubator: holding her skin-to-skin on your chest, your skin temperature increases or reduces in response to your baby. Your breasts will make the perfect milk for your child – special milk if she's premature, more thirst-quenching on a hot day, ebbing and flowing according to her needs.

If you generally 'live in your head', it might benefit you to holiday in your body for a bit. See what it's like to feel it, rather than think it. To experience the sensation, rather than analyse it intellectually. I say this because much of birth and motherhood is a sensuous, body-led experience, rather than brain-led.

Doulas and midwives working together

Once I've explained the role of the doula, a common question is 'Isn't that a midwife's role?' Well, yes it is. But just because, ideally, a midwife should be providing social and emotional support as well as clinical care, does that mean there is no room for anyone else? Can a pregnant, birthing or new mother have too much love?

Doulas have always complemented and complimented the care the midwife gives. The word midwife means 'with woman'. In French, it is '*sagefemme*', meaning wise woman. Doula means servant. We all have our role, our place and our boundaries. We must be aware of the grey areas and mindful of all the actors in this play. We must always ask ourselves how we can make sure everyone feels respected and appreciated.

If you are a midwife reading this, never think that doulas see you as the enemy. You are our greatest friends, because you have the same aim – a happy, healthy outcome for mother and baby.

Your doula is always thinking about how you can get the best, most appropriate care. She wants to know the midwives, supervisors, obstetric staff and anyone else at the hospital who may have an impact on your experience. She may offer to introduce you to people who can help make your dreams come true. We are a team, with the same goals and aspirations. All that matters is that the mother, father and baby feel heard and loved, and that they are given choice and control. If someone appears not to want that for you, perhaps they aren't the right person to be caring for you.

Some 'c'-words

Your doula may talk about 'choice'. For some reason she wants you to have some. A question I often get asked is, 'Surely the doctors know best. Shouldn't I just do as they say?'

We live in a world of choice and I sometimes wonder if there is too much of it – especially when I'm in the supermarket or flicking through the TV channels. But what has this got to do with childbirth? After all, having a baby is hardly comparable to buying a car or choosing new wallpaper. How can you make a selection when you know nothing about any of the options?

Most women, after seeing that thin blue line, are catapulted to a place where they don't speak the language, all the rules seem different and the only option is to cling to any life raft that is offered. It can be comforting to be led by the hand through the corridors of pregnancy and birth. They don't see all the other possible routes or the doors that could be opened. The doctors are the experts, right?

So, do we have the power, right, or liberty to choose? Women are denied this right, because how can they choose something they don't know exists? Your caregivers should be giving you choice – for these reasons:

1. There is almost always an alternative or an option to do nothing.
2. Because you have autonomy over your own body.
   You own yourself and your baby and you get to choose who does what to you and your bits and pieces! This is a fundamental human right that we often overlook when it comes to childbirth. No one would ordinarily have the right, for example, to insert their fingers into your lady-parts without asking your permission, explaining why and stopping when you say so. Why should that be different now you're pregnant?

Making your choices for birth may be simple, complicated by numerous options or narrowed by health concerns for you or your baby. But there will always be a choice that feels preferable for all – the scenario that seems closest to your heart's desire. This is your maternal instinct and it deserves to be acknowledged.

'Informed choice' is enshrined in our medical system – a gold standard that all health care providers should aspire to, and which should be written into the very fabric of philosophies of patient care. Informed means that you have enough information and have understood enough in order to choose, or give consent.

But remember, there is almost always an alternative. It might be considered so 'out there' or risky as to be almost universally ignored or declined – but no one has the right to make that assumption on your behalf. As a competent, intelligent adult, *you* should be the one to survey the menu and choose your meal.

Freedom of choice, freedom of action, freedom to bear the results of action – these are the three great freedoms that constitute personal responsibility. Such responsibility feels very grown-up, and I don't blame people who feel the need for the security blanket of 'conveyor-belt care'. I do passionately believe, however, that being an active 'chooser' or a passive 'recipient' of care should be a decision that is the prerogative of the 'patient'.

At the end of the day, you're having a baby. That's parenthood. The choices you make for the birth are you flexing your parenting muscles in preparation for all the other choices and decisions you'll be making for your child in the years ahead. It's one reason your doula will offer you choices and try to help make those choices as informed as possible; to help you feel strong and capable.

And here's another c-word: control. If you feel in charge of your choices, respected and loved by those around you, and are given time to make the choices that feel right for you and your baby, the more in control of the whole experience you will feel. When parents are interviewed after childbirth, a sense of control seems to be one of the most important aspects of a positive experience. This feeling seems to protect against trauma and postnatal anxiety or depression. So control is pretty crucial.

> I mentioned to my doula that I'd really like to give birth in the water... The next time I saw her she had brought a couple of books with her. I hadn't really thought about reading a book about water birth because it seemed quite straightforward. But this book was amazing... it gave a beautiful explanation of why the water helps... It also touched on other aspects of positive birth that I had not been ready to discuss after my previous traumatic birth. It changed the course of my birth preparations and contributed to my amazing water birth. I wouldn't have even picked it up in a book shop... but my doula knew exactly what I needed to read.
>
> Miriam MacMillan

Once you have painted a picture in your mind of how you'd like to have your baby, it can help to put those wishes and preferences down on paper. Your doula will encourage you to write your 'birth wishes' down. This helps the midwives caring for you on the big day get up to speed on what you want. Even if your maternity notes have a 'tick-box' birth plan page, this will only cover the bare minimum. Your own words are much better at expressing your hopes and fears, and give the staff a sense of who you and your partner actually *are*. I always think of it as like being invited to dinner. It would be very rude of me not to tell my hosts I'm vegetarian. Likewise, the maternity staff, whether you choose home, hospital or birth centre, will be helped by knowing a little about you so they can serve up dishes that will fit the bill.

I started Lamaze birth preparation classes wanting an elective caesarean. I left confident in the natural process and knowledgeable in my options for birth. I started to believe I could birth my baby and opted for a home birth.

Lisa Ramsey

If you are making 'unusual choices', the birth wishes document may take on a little more importance. Today's maternity services vary wildly from hospital to hospital and from consultant to consultant, so your 'bizarre' choice in Sudbury may be pretty normal in Surbiton. If you are having twins, or are pregnant after having a caesarean last time, you may find that you appear to have fewer choices. But with the support of your family, your doula and supportive medical staff, dreams can come true and birth choices you never thought possible can become a reality.

My doula introducing me to Ina May Gaskin's Guide to Childbirth *started me on the journey from wanting a hospital birth with an epidural to a homebirth...*

Sophie Messager

Birth rights

I believe you have what we in the birth world call 'birth rights'. These include your unalienable right to have the final say on what happens to your body and your baby. You get to choose where you have your baby and in what way. Every piece of advice or recommendation from a health professional, friend or family member is a kind offer that you can decline if you wish.

Some people who work in maternity care believe that you

have to be persuaded to take the safest, most appropriate course and that women, if left to their own devices, will do crazy, dangerous things. This is wrong on two counts. The first is that all the evidence suggests that when parents have access to all the information, they make safe and sensible choices. The second is that the practitioner giving the recommendation does not have access to all the pertinent information, so they don't always *know* what the best course of action is *for you*. Weighing up risks and benefits is something you have to do in partnership with your medical caregivers. The doctors may believe that a c-section would be the least risky course of action, but they don't have to come home with you afterwards and look after your two under-fives and a new baby. Another doctor may guide a mother towards vaginal birth because of pressure to bring the c-section rate down, without understanding her personal reasons for wanting an elective caesarean.

Your personal preferences, social situation and instinctive knowledge about how you want to give birth, matter. Your doula cares about you taking charge of your experience because we see the whole picture: your life and how this baby will fit into it. That's why we tell you you're *allowed* – because you are. And it's important.

I know some awe-inspiring health professionals. They would never coerce anyone into a course of action that didn't feel right. They truly understand informed decision-making and the need for mothers to give proper consent for any procedure. But all doulas have also witnessed practice that contributes to parents feeling upset and traumatised.

There is a turning-point coming: doulas, midwives and obstetricians are bearing witness and calling for change. It's fast becoming obvious that the current rate of interventions, the damage they cause and the financial consequences is not sustainable.

The last few years has seen the formation of organisations like Birthrights, Human Rights in Childbirth and The Roses Revolution, to complement the work of established organisations like the Association for Improvements in Maternity Services (AIMS). I have started the #feministbirth campaign and doula colleagues have created the Positive Birth Movement and Tell Me A Good Birth Story, which are spreading positivity and support around the world. Online breastfeeding support like Dispelling Breastfeeding Myths is creating new community and spreading reliable information. Doulas are involved in all these movements.

If you are pregnant reading this, I don't say this stuff to scare you. If I was your doula I'd be doing everything in my power to enhance the relationship of trust and partnership you have with your midwives and doctors. I firmly believe that everyone you meet has your best interests at heart. What I also know from over a decade of watching maternity services in action is that the service is increasingly not fit for purpose. We cannot continue to force pregnant women into large, centralised hospitals, treating them as disasters waiting to happen, piling them onto conveyor belts and pushing them through a system that is staffed by people who feel under-appreciated, underpaid and overworked.

We cannot punish staff for disagreeing with the status quo or bully them because they go against protocol. Maternity staff do good, every day, in a system that has been under-resourced for decades. Despite the Government knowing that something is deeply wrong with the system – proven by our skyrocketing caesarean rates and shocking breastfeeding statistics – there seems to be no will, political or otherwise, to create real and lasting change.

The chances are you'll meet some fabulous, kind, skilled people. But just possibly you may meet staff who are at the end of their tethers. Having someone around, with no other agenda than your own comfort and happiness, might just make a difference to how you feel as you progress through your pregnancy.

Birth rites

What are birth rites? This is about you designing your own pregnancy, birth and babymoon rituals. I know a lot of the women I support yearn for something they can't quite put into words. For many of us, I think, part of what is missing is our female tribe. We have the modern 'baby shower', but where are the fairy godmothers with wishes and gifts for the mother-to-be? Your social circle should be your strength, source of love, encouragement and trust in your abilities.

Increasingly, mothers are asking for 'mother blessings', sometimes facilitated by their doula. This is a time to bring your circle of friends together and for them to bestow gifts on you – more usually symbolic gifts to give you strength while you labour and hands-on blessings like massage or healing. This can all sound a little 'new age', but think for a minute about how it feels to have your best girl friends and favourite female relatives around you. We are a tribal species; the strength and courage we derive from each other is tangible. I've seen with my own eyes how a bracelet of beads made with donations from a circle of friends helps women in labour. It is as if all those kind women are in the room, urging you on, believing in you. I don't care how many people roll their eyes – if something helps a mother then it gets a thumbs-up from me.

Your birth rites might be anything you choose – from where you choose to labour, what you want to do, or look at – from a vision board or affirmations stuck on the wall, your hypno CD playing in the background, the use of essential oils, water, massage, music, dance or getting smoochy with your partner. It might be how you choose to welcome your baby, what you do with the cord and placenta or how your want to arrange the first few days and weeks of her life. It might also include choices you make as new parents – where your baby sleeps and how you transport her will all figure on your radar at some point. Birth rites are more than ceremony and ritual; many of them are practical, useful and add to your sum of health and happiness if freely chosen. Many will have proven benefits. The point is that you are the creator and everyone else will bow to your wishes.

The last days – ripe and ready

During pregnancy, your doula is there for you. You'll meet her a few times, forge a relationship and she will get an idea of your hopes and fears. Hopefully, you begin to look forward to the birth.

Then, unless you have a fixed date for your birth, we wait. Sometimes we're surprised by an early arrival. But more often than not, we wait. These days can be challenging, especially if you're feeling heavy, impatient and chasing around after other children. It can seem pointless – what are we waiting for? People around you may tell you how enormous you are and usefully predict that you're about to pop any minute, or make jokes about how many babies are in there. Her head might be pressed right down onto your bladder, making you feel like she's almost out – why doesn't she just get on with it?

Each day your baby matures a little more, readying her for life outside. Every Braxton Hicks contraction helps line her up so she can slip out easily. Every moment of rest or reflection readies you for what is to come, and is another step in your psychological transition. It is a time when the world stops, but radical change is taking place, imperceptibly, for you and your baby. Many mothers find it helps to try to honour these days, to mark them in some way. It will be the last time you and your partner are just a couple, or before your child(ren) get a new sibling and the family dynamic changes. The mothers I support who glide most easily through this time are the ones who decide that they won't fight it. They stay in the moment; my shorthand for this time is 'knitting and napping'.

Just as all ovens and all cake recipes vary, your baby will come when she is cooked. We can weigh and measure almost everything in this modern world of ours, but we have not yet cracked all the mysteries of pregnancy. Savour these last moments.

What is your doula doing during these waiting days? Being 'on call' is no mean feat. While carrying on the daily routines of children, seeing other clients and keeping our hearth and home ticking over, more than half our mind is on you and one hand on our mobiles. Our families and friends get used to us saying, 'Yes, I'll be there, babies permitting'. We don't drink, eat garlic or strong-smelling curry or wear perfume, and we go to bed early just in case. We pretend everything is normal – one doula friend of mine goes to the theatre when on call, and never seems to get called away mid-act. But large parts of our normal lives are cleared aside to make space in our hearts and minds for you. When I come home from a birth my husband says 'welcome home' – we both know he means more than just my absence for the actual birth.

A doula called Sally sums it up beautifully and famously in *Doula!*, a film made by Toni and Alex Harman:

> *A call in the middle of the night is not going to make me tut and roll my eyes; I'm going to be unbelievably excited.*

So never worry about bothering us. Waiting for you is our heart's desire and *raison d'être*.

Last-minute curve balls

Not all of us can calmly savour the last days of waiting. Sometimes health concerns can rear their ugly heads towards the end. Sometimes pregnancy continues for longer than the medics are happy with. This is quite common, especially in first-time mothers. There is a mountain of evidence showing that women are usually much less satisfied with their birth experience if they are induced. The use of pharmaceutical pain relief is statistically higher in these births and data increasingly show much higher use of instruments and c-section. Given that we routinely induce around 27 per cent of first-time mothers in the UK, it makes sense for you to have information about the pros and cons of routine post-dates induction. I usually point clients towards Sara Wickham's writings – she is a midwife who writes for AIMS.

I'm a very superstitious doula; I always think that, just as if you take your umbrella out with you there will be glorious sunshine, if you know about this stuff in advance, you won't need it.

Other concerns in the last part of pregnancy include amniotic fluid levels, the size and position of baby and your iron levels. As with anything else, I'd always say that knowledge is power. So question, ask lots of people for their opinion and make decisions based on the benefits and risks of the course of action on offer, after looking at the alternatives and considering what might happen if you do nothing at all. Your gut instinct will usually serve you well and you will know what to do.

Your baby is coming, waiting in the wings for her grand entrance. She knows how to be born, if we can just listen.

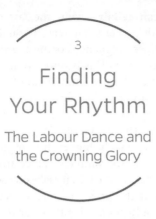

3

Finding
Your Rhythm

The Labour Dance and
the Crowning Glory

Labouring at home – all births are home births

Very few of my clients go into labour 'out of the blue'. There's usually some warning; a show, some light cramping, a row with the other half… and usually I get a text or two in the run up so I know to get everything organised in case I get a call in the middle of the night. Every so often though, I get a call and all I hear is loud mooing and a rasping, imperative '*Come now*'. It's those calls that make me wish for a Tardis and be thankful my bag is packed, my sandwiches made and my clothes chosen. In eleven years I've missed three births. They were all second or third babies that came in less than an hour.

It wasn't me being at the birth that was the important thing for those women. It was being there to help them recover from the shock of a very swift birth, tidy up, feed everyone and be a calm, smiling face after the drama of a whirlwind labour. I'm a great believer that things usually happen for a reason.

So if you're wondering about when to call your birth doula, I'd say just trust you'll know. Many of us spend time wondering 'Is this it?' You might have had a few days of little runs of contractions and assume it's all going to stop again. I once had a client who got to 8cm thinking she had an upset tummy – not a dreadful way to approach labour; it can be a little harder when you're focusing on every surge and intent on progress. Stay with people you love and trust, with as much privacy as possible, and send away anyone who makes you feel observed – a watched pot never boils!

A great tip is to try to distract yourself with anything that will help you deny you're in labour until it's absolutely undeniable! Resting/sleeping, eating and drinking and perhaps some relaxing strolls are about all that is expected of you right now. Once your labour has reached 'boiling point' it is much less likely that you'll go 'off the boil' if you go to hospital or strangers walk into the room.

If you fancy a chat with your doula, call her. It doesn't matter where you are in labour, if you think you might like the sound of her voice or her presence, call her. She doesn't care if it's 'too early' – she can always go away again once you no longer need her. She won't be resentful; it's part of our job.

Once you're a mum, you'll 'get' how your doula manages to reply to your late-night text, almost as though she was already awake, and look so zen at 3am. You'll understand how she manages to close her eyes for five minutes and appear to awaken totally refreshed. You'll totally identify with her habit of conserving her energy; curling up on your sofa and dozing while you don't need her physical support but merely her presence. Like any mum, she sleeps with one ear and one eye open. Sometimes we are completely awake but in a deep state of relaxation; the skills we suggest for labour are just as useful for your supporters. Unlike midwives, doulas don't go off shift, so we must pace ourselves. But if you need something of her, say her name and she will be by your side in a flash.

As far as the scientists can make out, your baby starts labour. A chemical conversation between the two of you signals she's ready for life outside and there's not a lot we can do to force her out before she decides it's time. If your body and your baby aren't 'ripe' it'll take a lot of shaking to get the apple out of the tree. That doesn't mean we can't do it if completely medically necessary, but if all is well with both of you, it'll probably be easier and less stressful if you wait for things to start in their own time.

Finding your rhythm: the labour

A common question is whether doulas meet clients at the hospital or go to their homes. I always aim to support parents at home first. Wherever you are planning on having your baby, the reality is that all births are home births. The hospital system is set up to support you during the last part of your labour (what the medics call 'established labour', from when your cervix is around 4cm-6cm open), so for many women the longest part of their labour will be at home. And home is usually the best and most pleasurable place for this phase. You can hang out in a place that is yours, feel comfy and private, eat and drink, sleep, watch TV, have a bath or shower and distract yourself with your activities of choice. Usually our own homes are where we feel safest and least inhibited and, given that this atmosphere is what our hormones need to flow nicely, home usually helps labour progress smoothly and effectively.

Getting your head round the fact that you will probably be labouring at home for a while, and that therefore it might be sensible to prepare, can make all the difference. I remember a postnatal client I had who was so traumatised by her labour that she needed treatment for PTSD. What she dwelt on most was her memory of being turned away from hospital. At home she was scared; she didn't know how to cope with the sensations, and her partner didn't know how to support or comfort her.

This is one of the ironies of modern maternity care: we are given a strong message that it is dangerous and reckless to birth outside the hospital, away from medical surveillance. Yet when we feel we are in labour and head for the 'safety' of hospital, many of us are turned away. If we go home and accidentally have the baby on the living-room carpet, we are praised by the medics for being 'good' birthers, yet if we plan to give birth that way, we are often discouraged and accused of taking risks.

While we continue to give conflicting messages to women about where and how to labour, it is no surprise that parents feel confused and abandoned. They not only lose confidence in themselves and their ability to make decisions, but can also lose faith in their caregivers. My job as a birth supporter and advocate is to try to shield parents from being caught in the crossfire between those who believe birth is risky and those who believe all women can do it without help.

The reality, as always, is not black and white. *Most* women, given a loving, supportive environment, which is warm, safe and private, will birth without trouble. But some women and some babies need help. Wanting help and not getting it can be just as traumatising as dreaming of an intervention-free birth and ending up with drugs and instruments. I think it's time we got realistic about birth and started talking about supporting every woman, instead of making sweeping generalisations.

But let's get back to early labour, hanging out at home. This is when you find your rhythm, trying out the coping strategies and techniques you might have practised during pregnancy. This is when women understand why antenatal teachers, doulas and midwives go on about rhythm – it really helps. It's not uncommon for a doula to be told that before she arrived the pain was getting overwhelming, but that as soon as she appears, the contractions are much easier to cope with. We do not work magic, but we will immediately encourage a woman who is rooted to the spot, tensing up against the sensation, to let go and move, sway, spiral her hips or 'dance', shifting weight from foot to foot. Your baby is moving, rotating, descending. She needs soft, fluid, moving tissues and bones to work with, not a static, rock-hard environment. So do the 'doula-hula' and dance your baby out.

Don't forget to eat, drink and go to the loo. Labour is a job that, once it gets going, requires all of your attention. And like any task that needs focus, it's easy to forget those little messages that tell us we're hungry, thirsty or need a wee.

Women often find something repetitive to do during contractions. It can be anything from pacing, counting, singing a song or chanting a mantra or affirmation. There have been a few times when I've been invited by the woman to join her in her chanting – I feel a little sorry for people who walk into the room to be greeted by a doula, mum and dad rocking and chanting or, on one memorable occasion, singing nursery rhymes! I've known mums squeeze stress balls, bang my pilates balls together, pick at the hole in her husband's t-shirt (that was me!), count the tiles in the shower, separate a box of tic-tacs into separate colours and cut their own hair in front of the bathroom mirror. Whatever it is, if it feels good, do it. It's not mad, it's not crazy; it's just your brain and body doing what it needs to do.

At home you find the strategies that you will take with you to hospital, if that's where you're going. You might find smells you hate and love, what touch you like or need, what you like to look at and listen to and ways to help you silence that chattering neo-cortex.

Hopefully you'll have got into a rhythm of eating what you fancy, drinking regularly and going to the loo. I'm a big fan of the loo. It helps bring on good, effective, opening contractions, feels comfy for most mums and encourages you to let go and relax your pelvic floor. If you sit the wrong way round on the seat, you really open your pelvis and can rest your head on a pillow on the cistern. Someone can massage your back if you want. The toilet is usually the smallest, most private room, perfect for the flow of that marvellous labour hormone, oxytocin.

If you're planning a home birth, so it goes on. You may move from room to room or get in your pool and when you feel it is time to call a midwife, you do. And she comes. In the majority of cases, contractions get closer together, longer and stronger until you can feel the baby coming down.

Our doula was incredibly helpful during the labour! She answered any queries I had and she was available as soon as we asked her to come to our house. When I asked for extra support with the surges she knew all sorts of tricks: acupressure points to offer pain relief, hip squeezes, pelvic movements, use of aromatherapy, homeopathy... These really helped! With each surge our doula would dig her knuckles into the acupressure points on my back and my husband would squeeze my hips or rub my thighs... It felt like brilliant teamwork and empowered my husband to be an integral part of the birth... I feel every woman would benefit from this kind of motherly love and support.

Jane Parsons

When baby comes in a hurry

During pregnancy most women spend time imagining how and where they will give birth. Sometimes, however, babies have other ideas. We have all heard stories of women giving birth in unusual places. The media revels in stories of husbands or passing members of the public 'delivering' babies who cannot wait until the mother reaches the haven of hospital. We have medicalised birth so much that childbirth is seen as something that takes a long time and needs lots of intervention. When women give birth quickly and efficiently, it takes people by surprise.

One of the problems with the idea that childbirth is dangerous and only appropriate in a medical setting is that some women attempt to get to hospital when they might be safer staying put. I am regularly surprised when I speak to mothers with a history of fast birth, who live more than a few minutes' drive from hospital, who are advised to come in. The possible outcome of this blanket advice is babies being born on the side of the road, or alone at home without a midwife. It seems to me that the risks of birthing in inappropriate places (babies getting cold, for example) or a mother feeling traumatised by birthing alone, are greater than putting plans in place for a home birth.

Even first-time mothers sometimes birth quickly. Despite a mainstream cultural view that fast birth is a 'good thing', the super-quick dilation and descent of the baby usually means that a woman's inbuilt pain-relief mechanisms don't have time to build in proportion to the intensity of the contractions. Fast birth can be a very wild ride indeed, without a moment to catch the breath or stop to think. As a doula, I think that all parents benefit from spending a few minutes during pregnancy imagining that kind of scenario and talking through what they might do. I want parents to know that if birth is happening fast, the likelihood is that everything is OK. It's alright to trust their instincts about attempting the journey or staying where they are and calling for support. Sometimes a midwife will make it in time, and sometimes maternity staff will call on paramedics to provide medical back-up. Often a partner or the mother herself catches the baby. It is the mother who 'delivers' the baby. Anyone else present who may find themselves with a baby in their hands has merely caught the baby – they have prevented the baby falling on the floor. While that is an enormous honour, it is nothing special – the mother has done the work and deserves the credit. And that goes for any type of birth.

The most important things are to keep the baby warm by placing her skin-to-skin with the mother and leaving the cord alone. Birth in an unexpected situation can be an enormous shock, which can make the mother shake uncontrollably, increase adrenaline levels and slow the birth of the placenta. Making sure she feels safe and warm is crucial.

Making the move

If you're planning to go to hospital or a birth centre, when should you go? Much thought and worry accompanies this question. Many parents say they've been told it's when the contractions are coming every five minutes and lasting a minute. But I've known women to be pushing out their babies with that pattern of contractions, and some who haven't yet started to open. A better guide is you. Your feelings, your instincts. The sensations of labour are much, much more than numbers and timings. Sorry, it's another of those piece of string questions: you will just know.

Getting in the car because you're scared, because the traffic might be bad, because *you* don't know what to do with yourself at home or because your mother/sister/neighbour says you should are not the best reasons to leave your home. If you are going because you need to be where your baby is coming out, then now is the right time. Your partner and doula can make suggestions for ways to comfort you at home, ask what you need and help you get ready to go. The midwife on the end of the phone can listen and ask questions and help you assess whether or not now is the time, but ultimately, it's your call.

Taking the birth centre or hospital transfer in your stride, and what if you don't want to go?

If you decide to move from home, a car ride is probably inevitable. I've heard lots of women say that the labour was perfectly doable until they got in the car. Sitting still, with a seatbelt on, with contractions coming regularly, is not fun.

How you get to the hospital will be up to you. Some people in cities will call a black cab – you get lots of room to move about and space for your bags. Remember to take a blanket or similar to put under you to protect the seats if your waters break dramatically and a bag or bowl in case you feel sick. If you're going in your own car, it might be an idea to leave the baby seat at home. It takes up loads of space and someone can easily come home for it after the baby is born. It's more important right now that you can find a position that is comfy. Lots of women find themselves kneeling on the back seat, either on all fours or leaning on the back shelf.

If you have a doula, she can be in the back with the mother, leaving the partner free to drive without distraction. Partners reading this – stay calm and take it easy. Road bumps and sharp corners were designed to torture women in labour. Take those extra slow.

Have a pillow to help you get comfy. For some women, something over their heads (or a blindfold of some description) and their favourite music or hypno-script on their headphones will diminish the stress of the journey and keep those labour love hormones surging nicely. Others will find that whatever they do, the journey results in a calming-down of the contractions. Lots of doulas can tell stories of walking into the labour ward with a mother who looks like a woman not in labour. Once you feel safe and private again, your contractions should return. And if they don't and it looks like you're in early labour, you can always go home again. I know it feels annoying to be sent home, but the midwives know that home is often the best place for your labour to really get going. However, if you know you need to stay, dig in your heels and be assertive, or find the hospital café. I've often found myself with clients in the hospital chapel – it's usually quiet and private and a great place to do some labouring, close enough to the labour ward to reassure the mother.

Make sure you know how to get to the hospital, an alternative route if there is a traffic jam and where to park your car. Having an idea how you might get into the building in the middle of the night might be useful too.

Yes, it helps your local midwifery team if they have a basic idea of how many women are due around the same time as you and roughly where they may like to push out their babies. That way, they can arrange staffing rotas. But when push comes to shove, if you change your mind about anything, at any time, all you have to do is pipe up. So if you've booked a birth centre birth but then can't face the idea of getting in the car, or are very much enjoying your home environment, then say so. Call a midwife; dig in your heels. Midwives are usually wonderful and will move heaven and earth for you if they can.

Likewise, if you've planned to stay at home, and you suddenly feel you need to go in, go. They're not going to tell you there's no room at the inn. If you've been evangelical all pregnancy about having a drug-free labour, but now desperately feel you need an epidural or a caesarean, explain how you feel and make it clear what support you need. If you've been looking forward to your elective for 40 weeks and now you are yearning for a vaginal birth, feel empowered, change your mind, be assertive, get the support you need, weigh up the risks and benefits and follow your heart. Spontaneous changes of mind can be scary, but they can make you feel invincible.

Settling in and making it home

When you arrive, you should be greeted by a midwife and made to feel at home as soon as possible. Different hospitals have varying admissions systems; you may be taken to a triage room to be assessed before being admitted, or you might be shown straight to the room in which you will hopefully give birth.

Since birth moved into the hospital a generation or two ago even healthy, normal pregnant women have become 'patients'. Some of us are happy with that approach, but an increasing number of us, if all remains normal, want to birth our babies with minimal interventions and interruptions from doctors. The symbol of the 'pregnant woman as patient' is the obstetric bed. It usually takes pride of place in the centre of the room and dominates the space. All our lives we have been invited to 'pop up onto the bed' by doctors and nurses. However comfortable you've been moving freely at home, it's amazing how strong the draw of the bed can seem in hospital.

It is deeply culturally ingrained that we give birth in bed, on our backs. The reality, however, is that babies need gravity and movement to come out and, just as importantly, mothers generally find lying on the bed very uncomfortable. Actually, let me put that another way; if you've ever lain on your back in strong labour, you could be forgiven for believing that the position had been invented to torture you.

The lithotomy position (lying on your back with your legs in stirrups) was invented for the benefit of those standing in front (the root of the word 'obstetrician' means this) so they could comfortably deliver your baby. It was not invented for you. A loving midwife will catch your baby while you stand, sit, squat, kneel on all fours or swing from the chandeliers – do what comes naturally and consider ignoring the bed unless you feel the need for it, or there is a clear medical reason.

If you end up in a consultant-led unit to have your baby,

but you are normal and healthy when you arrive, don't be frightened to rearrange the furniture. You can push the bed to the side and ask for anything you might need – a birth ball, a mat for the floor, or a bean bag, for example. As a doula, I sometimes go in and put my client's bags on the bed. It's a clear reminder that the bed is not for lying on if you'd prefer to stay active, forward-leaning and upright. Most beds are adjustable, so if it makes a comfy leaning post, raise it higher. If you fancy kneeling and leaning over it, bring it down as low as it'll go.

I always have a rebozo (colourful Mexican shawl) with me. I'll often lay one on the bed to break up the oceans of hospital white. My rebozo also sometimes gets hung at the window to keep out some light or brighten up a drab space. Your doula may have many useful rebozo tricks up her sleeve to help comfort you during pregnancy and labour, or help your labour progress.

You can stick pictures or affirmations on the walls, make the space smell like home with your favourite essential oil, unpack your picnic, move the furniture, use your own pillow and generally make yourself at home. The more you can feel like you 'own' the environment, the more likely it is that your labour will progress smoothly.

Some more 'c'-words and some 'f'-words too

Those yummy feel-good hormones (endorphins and oxytocin) are the chemicals that keep you serene, drive your labour and provide you with the tools to cope. They give you a sense of being linked in love and shared experience with everyone around you, and enhance your empathy and ability to read others' emotions. They keep you calm and blissed out – helping you get to that place doulas call 'labourland'. So some more 'c'-words for you are 'calm' and 'connection'. Anything that threatens that sense of equilibrium may cause you to make a little bit too much adrenaline or cortisol. These stress

51

chemicals can have an impact on your contractions. High levels of adrenaline can cause the three 'f's; making you want to fight, take flight, or freeze, none of which are particularly fun or conducive to a smooth labour. Oxygen-rich blood can be redirected away from your uterus and your baby towards your extremities. This can cause stress to your baby and take much-needed energy away from the muscles of your uterus.

Stress hormones are the product of another f-word: fear. Fear causes us to tense up and can increase our perception of pain. More pain equals more tension, and so on. So it's important to do everything you can to limit your fear. Learning about childbirth and how to ride its waves can really help diminish your anxieties. Being supported by the right people, in the right way, helps too. Sometimes finding your safe place will be what works for you – being completely alone for a while is perfectly acceptable. Your companions will guard the door.

It's also worth noting that high levels of adrenaline can slow or stop your contractions. This is Mother Nature's way of keeping you and your baby safe; if a tiger comes into your cave, you need to stop your labour and run away or wallop it over the head with a rock. Thing is, your primal brain can't tell the difference between a tiger and someone you don't know or like. Think very carefully about who you invite to your birth party and consider what each of them will bring to help you, rather than hinder you. And don't be afraid to banish people if they are getting on your nerves.

A doula's role is to be acutely aware of you, your feelings and what you may need to feel safe and loved and uninhibited. I try to care for a woman as though she is my own child, because I know that the love I feel helps tension to dissipate, encourages relaxation and helps the mother melt into the labour surges. I sometimes want to use the word surrender, but I know that is a very loaded word for many abused women. However you want to describe it, softening and melting into the surges, floating over the waves of labour, requires an ability to 'let go' and indulge in the sensations washing over you. If your inner voice is screaming 'no', experiment with changing that to a yes. How does it feel?

If you realise you've been flooded with stress hormones, it can help to try to discharge them. Marching on the spot can con your body into thinking you've 'taken flight', or squeezing a stress ball or banging two together can make it think you are 'fighting'. Once the stress has diminished, those lovely chemicals of calm can once again begin to drive your labour in the right direction.

Learning how to switch off the chatter in your head and sink into the sensations of your body is a skill for labour and life. Many antenatal education systems, techniques and workshops promise you the key to coping with birth. Whether they are yoga, Active Birth, breath-work, meditation/relaxation or self-hypnosis, they all teach you to do the same thing: step out of your mind and into your body. In the words of midwife Ina May Gaskin, we have to let our 'monkey brains' do it.

Having a doula... empowered me to conquer childbirth without epidural for the first time. I felt safe, I felt free to completely let go, be myself and do what I needed to do. At the most intense moment, just as I began to doubt myself, she looked straight into my eyes and said quietly 'just a little longer'. It was exactly what I needed to hear.

Lauren Mishcon

As this mother found, calm reduces pain. Using your breath and your mind (visualisation, affirmations or hypno-techniques) quietens the neo-cortex and helps you float off into a daydream state. Using your body to flow and move through the contractions without inhibition or tension helps you deal with their intensity and actually helps your baby navigate her way through the pelvis. Focus on keeping your jaw loose and your vocalisations low; your jaw and throat are intimately connected with your pelvic floor. Don't believe me? Try singing a high note or clench your jaw and notice what happens to the muscles of your pelvic floor. Now sing a low note, relax your jaw or blow 'horse lips' and feel what happens.

Working out how your birth companions can support you physically and emotionally will help too. Perhaps you need them to remind you to stay loose, move your hips and to bring you snacks, drinks and a cool cloth or a heat pad for whichever part of your body needs it, to close the door and switch off the lights and help you feel safe and private and uninhibited. These things seem small, but the science is clear; the right conditions promote straightforward birth.

As a doula, my job is to understand that the mother is an oxytocin factory and to do all I can to enhance her production of this famous love hormone. If I love her, help create a loving environment where her partner and family can show her their love too, where she feels safe and able to express herself, then she will be much more likely to birth, bond and breastfeed with ease.

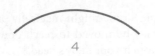

4

The Golden Hour

The New Family Meets and Greets and Eats

The final push

As you move towards being fully open, the contractions may be coming thick and fast: you can hardly catch your breath before the next one. That marvellous mixture of hormones has been building and building; you really are on another planet. All sense of time falls away. You may shake and shiver or worry that you can't do it. You may feel angry or frustrated or you may glide through transition without realising it is upon you. It's OK to express whatever emotions and sensations you're feeling right now.

The moment of meeting your baby is drawing closer. Some women will be fully open and get a rest for a while. This is a normal part of labour, called the 'rest and be thankful' phase. Eventually though, most women experience that undeniable sensation of the baby moving down. You may feel a pressure in your bum, like you need a poo. Your midwife or birth companion may tell you they can see the head and even how much hair your baby has. You may like to see for yourself, with a mirror your doula might magically produce from her birth bag. You may be moved to reach down and in with a finger or two to touch your baby's head.

Some women are calm and quiet at this point; others roar their babies out. There is no right or wrong. Some say the sensations of the second stage are different, that it's a kind of relief to feel that you are actually doing something with those surges of energy. This is when the adrenaline we've been trying to dampen down all through labour can actually be useful; I've known many worn out-looking women suddenly perk up when they realise they are beginning to push. That stress hormone can give us a little burst of extra energy, just when we need it. Sometimes women need an emotional purge around this time, or express a frustration or worry. I have been told some secrets at this point in the labour; don't worry, doulas are like priests when it comes to secrets.

Your doula and partner can support you physically at this time. You may feel the need to squat, with one support person on either side. You might need to hold your partner's hand or hang on a rope or rebozo. You might hear your doula's soft voice in your ear, reminding you to do what your body is telling you and that there is not long to go; your baby is nearly here.

There are as many different experiences of second stage as there are women: some swear they never feel the urge to push but the baby comes out anyway, while others are overcome with an overpowering, undeniable bearing-down sensation. Like a sneeze, it is a reflex that is impossible to ignore. Others find it takes a while to work out what's going on. I've known mums to be anxious, looking for guidance, and it can be tempting to give it. Perhaps that is the origin of well-meaning medical staff urging women to hold their breath, put their chins on their chests and push into their bottoms for the count of 10.

> *When my first child was born, the midwives told me*
> *that now I could push (as the head was crowning). All I*
> *remember saying (rather loudly) was 'are you INSANE?'*
> Fiona Willis

This 'purple pushing' (so called because it tends to make mums red in the face) can divorce mothers from the real sensations, in much the same way as if someone tried to tell you how to sneeze – it kind of scares it away. Breath-holding can result in less oxygen reaching your baby, as well as quickly tiring you out. Of course, you may have an epidural and not feel the urge to bear down. Or there may be concern about your baby and it's prudent to try to hasten the birth. Whatever the circumstances, it's useful to try to get as upright as possible – if you have an epidural, asking your support people to help you up and off your sacrum can make all the difference. Pulling on a rebozo or rope tied to the bottom of your bed or wrapped around a support-person's waist during contractions can help you sit upright and open your pelvic area.

Unmedicated mothers like to push in all sorts of postures – all fours, standing, squatting, sitting on the toilet or birthing stool or leaning over the side of the birth pool. Often they crave being upright and grasping hold of something. Some women instinctively adopt a position on their knees, leaning over the back of the bed.

I often suggest that home birth clients make a homemade potty-come-birth stool by putting some pipe-lagging around the rim of a bucket. This super trick facilitates many things – the mother can wee in it instead of struggling upstairs, others in the house can wee in it if the mother is labouring on the only toilet, or she can sit on it to push if it feels good. This bucket has saved me a few times when the need to pee has been overwhelming. I don't mind peeing in people's back gardens, but the neighbours may not enjoy the sight!

> *I was desperately trying to tell the midwives (they were in my front room, I was on the toilet) that I wasn't having a wee but was actually having a baby. I literally could not form the words as his head was crowning so I just screamed 'RING OF FIRE' as loud as I could. I'm afraid he still went down the loo head first, poor little poppet!*
>
> Trudi Withers Dawson

Your doula and birth companion will mop your brow with a cold cloth if you want it and give you sips of your favourite drink.

At some point the widest part of your baby's head will present itself at the exit. This is the moment when it can really help to S-L-O-W things down, to allow the tissues there to stretch, open, soften and let out the head without tearing. You may hear your midwife saying 'pant' or 'blow', but even if she weren't there, the chances are the sensation would stop you pushing and you would catch your breath for a minute, look up and find the eyes of a companion.

The birth hormones that have been building during pregnancy and labour are now reaching a peak. You are about as love-drunk, euphoric and blown away by the intensity of the moment as you'll ever be.

> *I remember looking at my husband, and as the wonderful hormones flooded my body, I was so happy I shouted 'I'M DOING IT, BABE! I'M DOING IT!!!!' He still laughs at that.'*
>
> Ashley Scott-Fisher

There's a moment, which seems to stretch into infinity, when the head is out and we are waiting for the next contraction, the head to turn and the first shoulder to be born. Some babies take some time and others are out in an impatient whoosh of gloop and blood, creamy vernix and amniotic fluid. They are a purple-grey colour for the first moments before they begin to breathe and turn pink. They may be screaming or be quiet and alert. Some are born in the bag. Watching the bag of waters balloon in the water before the head is born is like watching a mother lay a beautiful, mother-of-pearl egg.

Playing it out in theatre

No one disputes that the rate of surgical births, with over a quarter of all babies born by caesarean and more helped with instruments, is high enough to have created problems. While many countries in the world do not have adequate access to surgical birth, most Western countries seem to lack the resources to help women who want one maximise their chances of vaginal birth. There are no judgements attached to the way you have your babies. We know, however, that the health of a population of mothers and babies is optimised when the caesarean rate is kept under 15 per cent. Caesarean birth happens less often when women have a doula – we seem to have a beneficial effect – but that certainly isn't because we're telling women what to do.

We doulas inevitably support women having caesareans. I have supported elective caesareans, been present in theatre to witness ecstatic births and once held a woman's cold hand as her blood fell in puddles around our feet, holding my breath as the doctors saved her life. Thankfully this is a very rare occurrence in the UK, where giving birth is generally very safe.

If you have had your baby in theatre, your doula will be waiting for you. She may even be granted permission to come with you if that is very important for you. If your doula is your primary birth partner, she will be welcomed in theatre. If not, you may need to be assertive to make sure she can continue to support you both during a surgical birth. Most often though, your doula will be left in the birth room – she'll tidy up your possessions, reflect and maybe shed a little tear if she knows this wasn't what you wanted.

We hope that having loving support from all around you will allow you to bend with the wind and adapt to the new direction. However your baby comes out, it is your birth and you still have choices.

> *My clients were both very squeamish so once it was decided that a caesarean was needed they both asked me to go instead of the father. Thanks to the compassionate care of the obstetricians they allowed both the father and I to go in. His squeamishness vanished the moment his son was born and my being there gave him the confidence to step well outside his comfort zone and be there to support his partner and see the birth of his son. It was wonderful team work. The other time I went in to theatre was as a sole birth partner/doula at the end of a long induction. As the baby was born we had negotiated immediate skin-to-skin. The mother scooped the baby under her gown, placed her head under too and sang to her. I cried buckets!*
>
> Rebecca Schiller, doula

Most of the time, however, we are left to wait for your return. I'm usually ignored by the staff at this point. They have much more important things to be doing, so I'm not complaining. But it feels good when someone acknowledges the lonely, left-behind doula. I'll never forget the midwife who walked into the room with a cup of tea and a slice of toast and gave me a hug. She knew I had been there, without a break, for 48 hours. She understood how emotionally invested I was in my clients – and how tired! Midwives reading this book, please know – we really do love our clients. We know them well and if they end up with a caesarean that we know they didn't want, it hurts us too. On top of that, we might not have slept since… well, sometimes we can't remember when. If you see a sneaky tear, that's why.

The 'birth pause' – the moment of recognition

I remember one particularly beautiful water birth in the labour ward of my local hospital. The baby boy was born in his bag of membranes and he was guided up to the surface of the water by the midwife and handed to his mother. He solemnly looked up at his mother, the membranes still attached to his head like a bride's veil, floating out behind him on the surface of the water. Everyone in the room held their breath. The beauty of the scene seemed to stop time.

It is a heart-stopping moment. I'm not religious, but this moment is as close as I ever get to feeling the presence of a deity in the room. I never stop being surprised: oh wow, a person just came out of a person!

These days, most babies are instantly plonked on their mothers' chests. This is wonderful, but we really do go on one wild trip to birth our babies, and it takes a minute or two to come back down to earth. I've spoken to many women who remember not really being aware of the baby until they were fully 'present' after the intense rush of pushing.

Interestingly, it is often the fathers who laugh, cry or express extreme emotion at the moment of birth; the mothers are still on a crazy trip and need to centre themselves. If left to themselves, mothers will take a moment to look at the baby, then touch her and then finally scoop her up and bring her to her chest. Others have observed this phenomenon and named it the 'birth pause'. It is a moment to gather yourself, examine your infant and bring your child into your embrace at your own pace. It is a powerful and emotional moment for everyone in the room and I believe passionately that it is the first step on the most gentle, intuitive and organic transition to the world for the baby and an important way for the mother to integrate her transition to a new state.

One woman I supported suffered from an overwhelming anxiety that she wouldn't love her baby; worse, that she would be repulsed by her. Explaining the birth pause to her and reassuring her that she could greet her baby at her own pace did much to calm her fears. On the day of the birth, the midwife lay her baby on the bed and waited. Tears streamed down my face as I silently watched her first touch her baby with the tips of her fingers, then with her palms, and then finally scoop her baby up into her arms with a whoop of joy.

At this moment as the doula in the room, I step back. It is a moment for the family to savour. The midwife is keeping an eye on mother and baby. Perhaps your partner is there, enveloping you both with loving arms. The mother must touch and smell her newborn, realising she recognises the baby, like an old friend come to visit. As doula Mars Lord says:

> The best thing about the birth pause is when everyone sits right back and mum, dad and baby fall in love with each other. You can feel the oxytocin rising and rising and a sense of the miraculous happening fills the room. The only sounds are of a new family forming. It is too precious to do anything other than stand in awe of its power.

When a baby is first born, for a while, it is neither here nor there. While her lungs may be expanding and those first breaths are being taken, the placenta and cord are still pumping oxygen-rich blood to the baby, protecting her through her transition to this world and making sure she has her full complement of her own blood. Researchers believe that if the cord is cut immediately, the baby may be deprived of over a third of her blood volume.

As a mother touches and holds her baby, as they gaze into each other's eyes, as they smell and explore each other's bodies, as they finally come together in the first nursing, the hormone of love is surging through both of them. It begins to form the first bond, setting a blueprint for a secure attachment that will last a lifetime. As the oxytocin peaks, it begins a new round of contractions, which begin to separate the placenta and expel it. Your birth is not finished until the placenta has been born. The same environment, the same hormones, the same need for privacy and warmth are necessary.

It's important the mother feels warm and private, so I'll wrap them in warm towels or blankets, making sure the baby is skin-to-skin with her mother, and retreat to make tea. A midwife's skilled and observant presence has been a great reassurance during the labour and is equally important as the placenta is born.

The birth of a baby is also the birth of a mother. The cocktail of hormones that flows round her body in late pregnancy and during labour continue their job the moment the baby emerges. They ensure the baby is alert, with dilated pupils so she looks as cute and lovable as possible. The mother-baby gaze ensures that the mother begins to feel a close connection with the child. These hormones ignite the 'lioness' within – fierce in her protective instincts, alert to the needs of the baby and familiar with her unique smell and the sound of her cry by around 24 hours after the birth. Fathers often report an instant bond, or say that it 'hits' them the first time they hold their child and gaze into her eyes. Fathers also often say how in awe they are of their partner – how strong and wonderful she was giving birth. This feeling can strengthen a relationship and bind the couple in ways they never thought possible. Fathers can, however, fall prey to trauma and unhappiness during or after witnessing a birth. I think society needs to be a little more understanding of the needs of partners.

For many parents, this overwhelming feeling of love and attachment is instant. For others the feelings blossom over the days and weeks following the birth. For a few, it takes longer. The important thing is that the parents understand there is nothing abnormal in the way they react to the birth of their child.

Much has been written about how a 'good' birth can be a firm foundation for parenthood. We all know that a woman who is an active participant in her birth, in control of the birthing environment and who pushes out her child under her own steam, unmedicated and fully 'in the moment', very often feels hugely empowered, ecstatic and with such boosted self-esteem that she is more able to cope with the rollercoaster ride of early motherhood.

However, I do feel that even if the couple don't wish to opt for a 'normal birth', or they don't get the birth they dreamed of, they can still come out of the process feeling strong and whole, with the skills and strength they'll need to see them through. Research consistently comes up with the same results: women who feel in control, able to make informed decisions and who are respected and treated kindly, feel mostly positive about their births. Most of that comes down to how people around you communicate.

A client of mine chose to plan a home birth after a caesarean. After pushing for a long time, she knew she needed to go to hospital for some help. This was a big step because her first birth had left her traumatised and those emotional scars still ran deep. On arrival, I ran to find a midwife I knew, to ask her if she could find us the most gentle and respectful doctor she knew. She smiled warmly and reassured me – a lovely registrar was on shift.

When he entered the room he knelt at my client's bedside. I had never before seen a doctor do this. He touched her gently on the shoulder, looked her in the eye, said hello and asked, 'What do you need from me? How can I help?'

The mother told him she thought her baby was stuck and that she needed a caesarean. He quietly asked if he could examine her. With her consent, he performed the quickest, gentlest and non-invasive vaginal examination I have ever witnessed a doctor carry out. He nodded and told her he thought she was perfectly right: her baby needed some help to be born. My client looked at me. I knew she wanted me to explain her preferences for a surgical birth. I stepped forward and offered him her birth wishes document. He smiled, waved aside my proffered piece of paper and gestured for me to join him on the other side of the room. He asked me to explain what she would like and I explained her preference for a 'gentle caesarean', with immediate skin-to-skin. He was very respectful of me too, thanking me for helping him understand how she wanted it to be and expressing how much he loved facilitating caesareans this way.

He walked across to the mother again, smiling, and said, 'Come on, let's go and have a beautiful birth'.

Here's the client describing the birth of her baby:

I was prepped, the operation began, and once the screen was lowered, [the doctor] eased my baby boy's head out. We were transfixed. The room was completely silent, no one touched him. He looked around, moved his eyes, then slowly his body emerged from my abdomen. It was truly magical to watch. [The doctor] lifted him from my body and onto my bare skin. He was covered in buttery

> *vernix and throughout the rest of the operation I stroked*
> *his silky skin; he rooted around, cried a little, I held him*
> *constantly. It was so gentle and respectful, Nick and I*
> *were in tears. The theatre staff were buzzing about the*
> *operation – I was curious, surely they did this all the*
> *time? The anaesthetist explained how he'd administered*
> *syntometrine and my womb had contracted and*
> *squeezed the baby out. Wow!*   Rachel James

I include this story in detail because I think it exemplifies how little things can make an enormous difference. This doctor was gentle, respectful, communicated clearly, asked for permission, and remembered the parents are the centre of the story. And he didn't forget that the birth of a baby is always beautiful, always sacred, never work-a-day. I could have kissed him.

Whether it's a smooth, uneventful home birth, or an emergency situation, all parents deserve to be treated with kindness and respect and never coerced or pressurised into making decisions. Doulas are witnesses. We see instances of loving care all the time. Sadly we sometimes witness care that is unkind or even brutal. Thankfully, the powers that be are starting to wake up to the fact that obstetric violence is a real phenomenon, thanks in part to obstetricians like Amali Lokugamage, author of *The Heart in the Womb*, who are teaching student doctors about human rights in childbirth.

The third stage of labour – a piece of cake?

At some point, your doula will ask you about your preferences for your baby's first moments. How and when will you cut the cord, tie or clamp it or not cut it at all (lotus birth)? How might you birth your placenta and what might you do with it afterwards? Whatever you choose, the important thing is that this third stage of labour is respected and honoured.

We have fallen into a cultural norm that treats the placenta, which means 'flat cake,' as clinical waste, which seems rather odd, given what a crucial role it has played in your baby's development. It is, rather, a 'play-centre' – a place of joy, a thing of life and nourishment. It has been the centre of your baby's world. In some cultures, it is known as the baby's 'first mother' or 'older sibling'; it is honoured and disposed of in a ceremonial way.

Until recently, we thought the womb and placenta were completely sterile. We now know that life in utero is not entirely microbe-free. In fact there are 'good bacteria' in there, beginning the formation of your baby's immune system. Once your baby is born, her microbiome will continue to be colonised by bacteria in your vagina, on your skin and in your colostrum. If you are having your baby by caesarean, there is some research being carried out to find out whether babies born in this way benefit from being swabbed after birth with a cloth that has been in the mother's vagina. In this way, the baby is exposed to the right bacteria for optimal immune system development.

As a doula I have supported women who have begged the midwife to whisk the placenta away without it being seen, women who have wanted to keep it and bury it under a rosebush, make a print of it on paper (it makes an attractive 'tree of life' picture) or cook it and eat it (now there's dedication from a vegetarian doula as I fry your placenta up with some onions!). I have also made fruit smoothies with a thumb-sized piece of placenta and put the rest in the fridge ready for encapsulation (dehydration into capsules for later consumption) or tincture (a small piece of placenta in pure alcohol). Like all other choices my clients make, what I think is irrelevant. What is important is that parents are making choices about what to do with their own body parts and benefiting physically or psychologically from those choices. The placenta is full of vitamins, minerals and stem cells, for example, which could be beneficial to a postpartum mother. There is certainly no evidence of harm. And I have noticed a positive effect on milk supply when mothers have consumed their placenta.

I have also supported a mother's choice for a lotus birth. This is when the cord is not cut at all. The placenta is contained in something like a muslin bag and is salted and sprinkled with herbs daily so it dries and doesn't smell. The cord shrivels quickly and usually falls off the umbilicus within just a few days. Some people choose lotus birth for spiritual reasons, but there may also be emotional and social reasons – for example, the prospect of meeting the placenta may keep unwanted guests away for a few days while you recover from the birth.

Meeting and greeting

However your baby is born, the optimal place for her as soon as humanly possible is skin-to-skin with her mother. Skin-to-skin helps her transition gently to this dry world of heavy gravity and loud noise. Your chest is her new womb: as close as she can get to what has been her home for the last nine months. Her breathing, heart rate and her temperature are regulated: if she is cold, your body sends blood rushing to your breasts and chest to warm her. If she is too hot, the opposite happens, quickly and seamlessly in response to your baby's needs. Just like a kangaroo joey in her mother's pouch, a newborn thrives on her mother's chest. And if, for whatever reason, the mother's chest is not available, then the other parent's chest can serve. In an emergency, at the behest of the mother, we doulas have been known to stand in.

Sometimes women don't want immediate skin-to-skin.

The idea of holding a wet, slippery baby can seem repugnant. So if you want to be presented with a nice clean parcel, then state that on your birth wishes document, tell your doula and have her remind the midwife just before the birth.

Every so often, a baby has to be taken to special care. Your ecstatic moment is stolen from you by circumstance. This can be an agonising time, but your moment will come – that moment when, perhaps unobserved by anyone, you unwrap your baby and begin to become intimately acquainted with her body, taking ownership of her in a very primal way.

If you feel like sniffing and kissing her all over, that is normal. If you're petrified, that is normal. If you're so happy you think your heart will burst, that is normal. The cord may have been cut, but an invisible one remains, connecting your heart with hers. When she is close, the cord is slack and all is well with the world. When she is taken away, even if it is just across the room, that cord tugs on your heart. And it hurts. This is normal too. Keep her close if it makes you feel good, and if skin-to-skin feels good, consider leaving her undressed for now, and enjoy how it calms you both into a state of dream-like almost-meditation.

What is your doula doing while you meet your baby? There is always so much to do; tidying and washing up and preparing food and drink. There might be older children to care for. She may offer to help you to the shower, or clean you with a warm flannel. She wants to make sure your partner is OK, too. She'll be there with a hand to hold while the midwife checks your perineum. She won't leave you until she's happy you're OK or you kick her out. But she'll come back. You just have to call.

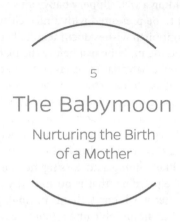

5

The Babymoon

Nurturing the Birth of a Mother

As you explore your baby's body, counting fingers and toes, smelling the top of her head and staring into her eyes, you will be blissed out on your own chemicals. Those hormones will be getting to work contracting your womb back to its normal size, slowing your bleeding and readying your breasts to eject milk.

After the birth, I love watching the baby rest quietly and then, when ready, begin to root around to find the breast – using a combination of smell, sight and touch, you and your baby wriggle together until everyone breathes a sigh of contentment as the baby latches on and begins to suckle. Another surge of oxytocin; one that is tangible in the room! This moment marks the beginning of your babymoon, a time measured out in milk and blood and the various colours of baby poo.

We all bleed after childbirth – however we have the baby. You might never have paid much attention to your blood before if you've been using tampons, so the amount of lochia (bleeding after childbirth) can take you by surprise. One of its purposes is to signal when we can get back to our busy lives, so while it runs, rest if you can. I once noticed a woman pushing a heavily-laden trolley around the supermarket. She had a toddler and, from the shape of her stomach and the look of the baby in the seat in front of her, a baby who was only a few days old. She looked harassed and careworn and increasingly stressed by the loud antics of her toddler and the cries of her baby. Being very British, I didn't like to say anything, but when I came across her again in another aisle and saw bright red blood dripping down her leg I couldn't stand by. I made her go and sit in the café with her children and I finished her shopping and stacked it all on the conveyor belt.

Our culture apparently worships the female form, yet expects far too much from it. It's assumed we'll just carry on, hiding our biology and never complaining. Actually, you'll probably want and need to give your amazing body a rest after childbirth, whether you push your baby out of your vagina or if you have surgery of any kind. And by a rest, I don't mean a few days. In most cultures women are tended to, nurtured and supported in their mothering for at least a month. All other tasks are seen to, so they can concentrate on themselves and the baby. It's not necessarily about being closeted in the house, but it is about having the cares of ordinary life lifted from your shoulders.

I've been lucky enough to have clients from all corners of the globe. It seems that we British are particularly bad at looking after ourselves after childbirth, as opposed to, say, my Chinese clients, many of whom still 'do the month', resting and eating special foods.

Just as we mark a new relationship by cementing it with a honeymoon, new parenthood demands we take some time out. Honeymoons are a private time, usually uninterrupted; time spent in bed, skin-to-skin contact, gazing at our lover, bathing in oxytocin. A babymoon is very similar!

Part of this pause after childbirth is about getting to know your postpartum body: appreciating your new shape, exploring any new markings, working out your new superpowers and discovering any new limitations. It's a time not only to get to know your baby, but also to carve out a slightly new dynamic in your relationship with the baby's other parent. Their experience of childbirth has been an adventure too. Showing love and intimacy during the postpartum months can be fraught with confusion or trauma, scuppered by tiredness or physical soreness, but it can also be a time of joyful reconnection and fruitful celebration of your fecundity.

So many aspects of our culture seem to try to make having a baby a minefield of complication and conflicting advice. As first-time parents, we are encouraged to believe that babies are a different species or even a machine that, with the right manual, will run smoothly. We are sold the idea that we give birth to baby rabbits that we can put safely in a burrow and leave there for hours. The reality is, we are primates; we give birth to baby primates. And primates are a carrying species. That means your baby is born expecting to be 'in arms'. Once put down, her sharp senses ring the alarm, to call you back to gather her up. She doesn't know there aren't tigers waiting just outside the cave. Even in 21st-century Western countries, there are dangers that lurk when babies are not kept close to a caregiver's body.

Becoming a mother, or a mother again, can be a strange time. Elation, depression, exhaustion, confusion, bliss, pain, joy, love, anxiety, isolation, excitement, fear and anger are just some of the emotions I see on a daily basis. What makes it even odder is that this amazing, magical transition goes on in private; hardly anyone sees you growing those beautiful mama-butterfly wings. Hardly anyone sees how they unfurl or watches as they grow stronger and you begin to use them to fly. No one sees your early trepidation or those first test flights that resulted in crash-landings. What society sees are almost fully-grown butterflies, flitting about with ease and at least appearing to be confident.

Your amazing transition is almost entirely hidden, witnessed only by your partner (who is also in transition) and maybe your mother or your doula. Society has forgotten to be duly amazed; we have lost all sense of wonder at the process and neglect to honour and celebrate parenthood. You'll probably get some congratulations cards and, if you're lucky, friends might cook you a meal. I very rarely see mothers being worshipped. Think that's a bit of an over-the-top phrase? A mother has grown and birthed a person, rearranging all her internal organs, her brain and her breasts in the process. Physically, psychologically, spiritually and practically, her body and brain have been completely dismantled and remade. It might have happened hundreds of millions of times before, but each time is as sacred and miraculous as the last. When it happens to you it can be overwhelming, or easy, or anything in between; but you deserve the status of goddess, just for a little while.

> there's… so much pressure to appear on top of everything and coping. Thank goodness for breastfeeding and being able to go back to bed guilt-free with my baby and my toddler until it's time for the afternoon school run! My daughters are the only ones that see my wings. My eldest tells me I am queen of the fairies; I am honoured with this title and [am] learning to grow alongside my precious girls. For now that is enough.
>
> Abigail Todd

Given that you're recovering physically, rapidly learning major new skills, suffering from sleep deprivation and working out a completely new identity, it seems logical that most of the mundane tasks of everyday life might need turning over to someone else. A lot has been written about the basic needs of a newborn, but much less attention is paid to the parents. What do you need in order to enjoy your babymoon? What can a doula or your family do to ease the passage into parenthood?

Lucy and Tom were over the moon to be having a baby, but beset by fears that manifested themselves in a thousand and one questions every time we met. As we got to know each other, I learned a little more about why they were so fearful. Both had fractured relationships with their own parents: Lucy had lost her mother in early childhood and Tom had a difficult, troubled relationship with his mother and a father who was withdrawn and quiet. Both felt they wanted to parent in a different, more loving and responsive way, but they weren't sure what that would look like. They bought lots of books, each one contradicting the last. It took some weeks for them to begin to relax and trust themselves. What made the difference, they told me, was their doula, who constantly asked, 'What do *you* think?', 'How are you *feeling* about this?', 'What do you *want* to do?' and most importantly. 'Look what a marvellous job you're doing!'

Once parents have accessed their instincts, it is usually easy enough for us to show them that science mirrors life: intuitive, responsive behaviour is associated with improved outcomes for baby and parents. If you want evidence that your instincts are spot on, your doula will be delighted to point you in the direction of good-quality parenting research or evidence-based guidance. From Facebook to the Cochrane Collaboration, we doulas collect things that might interest you. I often think part of the definition of doula is 'collector', or 'curator'. We love to share, too, so if your doula doesn't have a signpost for you, she'll know someone who does.

A doula's tender gift is to sit by you. To accompany you as

you begin to find yourself as a mother. To walk the path with you. To watch approvingly as you learn to nurse your warm, rooting infant. We have time. Time to spend on you. Because your food and drink is time. It is measured out by nursing sessions, nappy changes, the sleeping and thinking about sleep and worrying about sleep, the awake and in-between dream-time. We watch as your baby lies in your arms. We see her body squirm and ache to reach your breast. We might translate this new, alien language and ask, 'Do you think she's hungry?'

We postnatal doulas are the keepers of secrets, the celebrants of your emerging rituals, cheerleaders, champions of mothers and fathers. We have faith in you. As the psychologist Dr Kathryn Newns says: 'Sleep deprived, frustrated, sometimes even angry, it can be easy to forget that the person who usually knows what is best for their baby and their family is you.' Yet we are asked questions every day. Here are some of the most common:

Shouldn't babies be left to cry to teach them to self-soothe?
How do you feel when your baby cries? If you feel unsettled, upset or anxious when you hear that sound, perhaps evolution has designed those feelings for a reason? What do you ache to do when you hear her? If you can't wait to swoop in and gather her up in your arms, surely those feelings can't be against nature? You are not a freak. In fact the power of touch is amazing – just as important as food for your baby's growth and development. Would you like everyone to ignore you when you cry with anguish, loneliness, tiredness or hunger? Or would you prefer loving arms and softly spoken words of comfort? Have you become spoilt and demanding? I ask these questions in a genuine spirit of enquiry to support parents to find the way that suits them best. Some parents find that, rather than fixing the baby, finding coping strategies to go

with the flow of their very normal baby is more beneficial to everyone's sanity.

Don't babies need to be put into a routine as early as possible?
A few of us do eat and sleep to a strict regime every day. However, most of us have quite large variations in our appetites from day to day, dependent on the time, the weather, our mood or hormonal state and many other things. What might be the health benefits to your baby or to you of demanding your baby eat and sleep to the clock, rather than to hunger and tiredness? Perhaps it might be more predictable for you – and I'm sure that as your baby grows he'll be more inclined to meet you halfway – but when small, your baby's needs are intense and very pressing! Babies only have needs. Everything she asks for, she needs. Later on, when she's older, you'll find she falls into patterns and rhythms and will probably crave more predictability. Right now though, she's a bundle of instincts, reflexes and needs, with no circadian rhythms of her own. She only knows how to ask you to meet those needs so she grows and develops.

Isn't it dangerous to sleep in the same bed as a baby?
I wonder how this question sounds to an Amazonian tribeswoman or a villager in sub-Saharan Africa. How do you imagine the vast majority of the human race sleep, even now? We evolved to sleep in close physical proximity to a caregiver. The nights are long and dark and full of predators, and human babies are vulnerable. Your baby was born expecting to be able to touch and smell you all night. Some babies are fine being next to you on a different sleep surface. Many are much more insistent on feeling you close. Some babies will only sleep prone on someone's chest for the first few weeks.

Your baby's oxytocin-fuelled emotions are intense. Your

body, your smell, your touch, day and night, are more than just exquisite pleasure – it is what makes life bearable for her. Why are we adults allowed the comfort and security of our loved-one's body next to us at night, but our much more emotionally vulnerable babies are consigned to a separate sleep surface?

I would never tell you where your baby should sleep. That is for you to work out for yourselves. As your doula I would, however, offer to help you understand your baby, to explain how she might be feeling and why, and offer you some information on the science of infant sleep. As the vast majority of parents will share a bed with their babies sometimes, accidentally or otherwise, you might as well know a little bit about how to do it without feeling petrified or guilty.

When anxious parents pace the floorboards with an unsettled baby and then sit down on the sofa when the baby falls asleep, or when mothers get up and feed in a chair, they risk falling asleep with the baby in an unsafe position. On the other hand, appropriate bedsharing in a breastfeeding family with no other risk factors has been found to present no more risk than cot-sleeping. The Infant Sleep Information Service, a service provided by Durham University sleep researchers, states:

> The most recent UK study (conducted between 2003 and 2006) found that smoking, alcohol use and sofa-sharing explained the risk associated with SIDS deaths that happened when babies were co-sleeping with an adult.

Do babies need a bath every day? Do I need to use bubble bath?
You can keep a baby clean the midwife's way, Grandma's way or your way. Baby will still be clean. (For your information though, a baby's skin is much thinner than ours, so more

chemicals can penetrate.) You can use a bucket, the sink, your bath, a baby bath or a bowl of water and a washcloth. Common-sense applies – unattended babies and water don't mix, so have everything you need to hand. A nice way to get babies wet is popping them in with you. Super-magic skin-to-skin cuddles and you both get clean and relaxed. What's not to love?

Am I normal? Is my baby normal?
Yes. Even if your circumstances are unusual. Even if you or your baby are facing challenges that are not run of the mill, you and your baby are going through the same process of adaptation. You, and your baby, will be experiencing many of the same emotions and learning curves as anyone else. My experience is that many parents have been given a warped view of what is normal. We are fed many lies – for example, that sore nipples are normal (more of that later) or that a 'good' baby sleeps through the night. Yet we know nothing of things that are actually normal, like the colours of baby poo, or that baby girls sometimes have a little period, or what newborn sleeping and eating patterns look like. If you can find a good antenatal teacher, they are worth their weight in gold. Pump her, or your doula, for as much information as you can.

All you learned about the power of oxytocin, that hormone of love, in preparation for your labour and birth, is just as useful now. Love, manifested in touch, eye contact, eating and drinking, gentle movement, soothing sounds, smells and tastes, is just as important now. High levels help you stay calm through the challenges of parenting, help you feel connected and emotionally invested in your baby, squeeze out your milk and support your body to heal and recover from the pregnancy and birth. Oxytocin in your baby will help her learn, grow and bond with her parents and find how she fits into the social structure of her tribe. Love, in its basic chemical form, is pretty much all your baby needs.

What do you actually do?
I'm afraid this is another piece of string question. Every baby, every family, every babymoon is different. Things are unpredictable: you may start off thinking you need lots of support but then things go swimmingly well. Or you anticipate needing an extra pair of hands for a couple of days while your partner is away, but then your baby has high needs, your toddler has a difficult transition to nursery and you're feeling the strain. I've provided support for just two hours – and for two years.

You and your doula probably won't know when you will birth, how you will birth and what kind of baby is coming to stay. We doulas have to learn to go with the flow and provide you with as much flexibility as possible. We also have to give as much bang for our buck as possible. I remember a single mother I met once, who wanted to spend her savings to have me stay all night to support her. I would have been happy to – I quite like night-doulaing – but I could see she would be fine without it if she had some time to talk through how she felt and explore some practical strategies for dealing with the nights. Three hours during the afternoon, a chat and a nap, and she was all set.

Your doula's aim is to nurture the dyad; allowing the two of you to fall into your rhythms and get to know each other. So she may feed you, or cook something up for you to eat with your partner later. She might have a skill like baby massage that she can teach you. She may be able to massage you, helping to ease the physical strains of childbirth and holding and carrying a baby. She might know the 'Closing the Bones' technique, which comforts your aching hips and back, and helps your pelvis close again after childbirth.

She may leave snacks and drinks scattered around the house for you. She'll be happy to do your ironing, push the hoover round or peg out your washing. We all have stuff we're happy to do and stuff we'd prefer not to, so do ask her.

She's constantly thinking ahead so you don't have to. Will there be something for you to eat once she's gone? Are you running out of nappies? Would the evening and night be easier if you had a nap now, while you have someone here to watch the baby? She will be thinking about you getting through the 'witching hour' (although why it's called that when it typically lasts all evening, I have no idea) when both you and your baby may be at your most cranky, your baby may be cluster feeding and your toddler needs bathing and putting to bed. That particular juggle may seem overwhelming at first, but your doula may set you up with a comfy sling and some tips for coping.

> *The relationship with your doula is very unique and special. They see you at your most exhausted, emotional and vulnerable, but it is so wonderful to feel such unwavering, non-judgemental support at that time.*
>
> Alison Lawrence

Debriefing – the power of narrative

If you were to peek through the window at a mum with her doula, it might look like nothing at all. New doulas often tell me how guilty they feel because all they did was drink tea and chat to the mum, then cuddled the baby while mum napped. But they are underestimating the power of this 'intelligent tea-drinking'. It means so much to be *really* listened to, *really* heard.

Doulas spend a lot of time listening to stories. Stories are our lifeblood as human beings; especially for women. When I sit with a group of women aspiring to be doulas and we share our stories, I am always reminded how therapeutic it is to share in a women's circle and how few opportunities we get to do it. When

I am working with new mothers, I sometimes listen to the birth story over and over. The telling and retelling crystallises the story; it takes on the form that will become the official, 'public' version. Witnessing the evolution of the story, and with it the progression of the mother through her psychological journey, is fascinating. Storytelling is truly healing.

The oral narrative has been how women have communicated, shared life's wisdom and lessons, given and received, since the dawn of time. Our sex was illiterate until very recently in history. But with the written word came a silence – we stopped telling stories as part of daily life. But our circles are coming back; red tents, storytelling circles and other female rituals and rites of passage mean that perhaps our ancient stories will not be forgotten. Our narratives, be they personal, domestic or about universal wisdom, female power and mystery, are vital. It is how we share our strength and step into our inheritance at each stage of our lives – from maiden to mother to crone.

Stories can be used for good or ill. Too often I read stories written by women who use their own experiences to belittle the choices or feelings of others. Our stories can be used by commercial interests to pit us against each other ('We know breastfeeding can be painful, so if you choose to move on, our formula is here to save you.') or to silence us ('All the other mothers are so grateful – just be happy you have a healthy baby.')

We need to nurture our storytelling. We must listen carefully for the morals of the tales and use our yarns to knit us together, creating something beautiful and useful, rather than tearing each other apart.

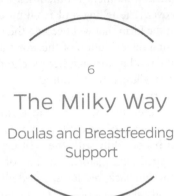

6

The Milky Way

Doulas and Breastfeeding
Support

Some doulas may know absolutely nothing about breastfeeding. Yet they have a magic way of creating a relaxed circle around the mother. They can project an air of security and supportiveness within which the mother feels free. They make it easy for her to give herself without fear to the relationship and the job of feeding. That's all some mothers need.

That quote is taken from a book called *The Tender Gift: Breastfeeding*, by Dana Raphael, published in 1973, in which the term 'doula' is first used. Dana was an anthropologist exploring the traditional practice, in some cultures, of new mothers being accompanied and supported through the initiation of breastfeeding by lay women from outside the mother's family. Dana always attested that the word doula came from the ancient Greek, meaning 'female servant', and that she'd found the reference in Aristotle. Here's what Dana thought about female companionship and support during birth and breastfeeding:

> *When a bottle-nosed dolphin gives birth to a calf, other adult females in the group help out by keeping her offspring afloat until he can fend for himself or until the mother regains her strength... these acts of caretaking increase the survival chances of that herd... in the case of human mothers, those who have some sort of 'mothering' from another person do well at breastfeeding, but those who do not can almost certainly expect trouble.*

Whatever the origin of the term, I think it does doulas good to remember that our roots are in supporting mothers to feed their babies. This thread in our work is important and powerful. And it is undeniable that we make a difference to the mothers, however they end up feeding their babies. The last Doula UK survey in 2014 found that '88% of women who had a postnatal doula were still breastfeeding at 6 weeks and 67% were still breastfeeding at 6 months. (This compares with 21% at six weeks and 7% at three months according to the Infant Feeding Survey of 2005 (Bolling et al 2007).'

Of course, it could be argued that doulas serve a small, well-educated, middle-class elite. This might have had a kernel of truth years ago, but these days doulas serve a broad spectrum of parents, right across the socio-economic scale.

Breastfeeding support as a doula gives me equal amounts of pleasure and pain: I am constantly enthralled by watching my clients step into their power as nursing mothers, and just as often appalled by the hurdles they encounter along the way. Today I visited a mother who was putting her baby to the breast only twice a day and bottle-feeding formula the rest of the time. She desperately wanted to be a breastfeeding mother – and nothing discernible stood in her way; she wasn't in pain, and had a good supply of milk, given how little she was breastfeeding. When she talked about how she was feeling and what she wanted, she explained why she wasn't nursing by telling me that she just felt like she 'didn't know how'. Her normal, as a nanny for many years, was the routine predictability of formula-feeding.

I asked a few doulas what makes such a difference to parents' experience of feeding when they have the companionship of a doula.

Because we have time, and we approach it with love and kindness and because we know how much it matters to our mummies and their babies.'   Lindsay Gale

Because we are invested. We genuinely care for these women and are willing and able to go the extra mile to support them in achieving their goals. As long as they want it we will be there, cheering them on, making sure that what they are doing is still what they want. We show them what good signposting and consistent support looks like.

Jo Gough

Sometimes it is just the sitting with a woman while she feeds, talking about anything or nothing, giving her the confidence to just be and learn her baby.   Mars Lord

Because we believe that women, their bodies, their breasts, work – and we offer the support, nurturing and love needed to make it so by allowing oxytocin to flow freely.

Vicki Williams

Of course, there are midwives, health visitors, breastfeeding counsellors and International Board Certified Lactation Consultants (IBCLCs) out there who are doing just this, and more. They work long hours, often in a volunteer capacity, supporting mothers as they start their feeding journeys. Some doulas are trained, qualified breastfeeding supporters too, but the particular role of the doula is to be that constant companion, the one who drives you to the support group, the one who rings the Lactation Consultant for you. The one who knows when things are normal and, crucially, when they are not. The one who doesn't have a badge or a uniform. The one who has the time to just 'be'.

A maelstrom of emotions whirls around in the early days but your doula is alongside you listening, sucking up some of that emotion and shouldering some of the burden. Sadly, these days, many mothers may not have anyone, other than their doula, who knows anything at all about feeding babies and who doesn't have strong opinions they feel compelled to share. More than that, your doula will probably have intimate knowledge of how you feel about feeding *your* baby.

> *My doula didn't pressurise me into making a feeding choice when I was unsure which way to go. When my son was born and I put him to my breast [I] instantly decided that I was going to bottle-feed and without any judgement my doula went into the kitchen and pressed start on the steriliser! I could not have been more grateful to have a doula who supported my choice without question 100%.*
>
> Lauren Derrett

In other words, a doula will be there for you, unconditionally, completely, whatever and whoever you are and whatever you do. And she will move heaven and earth to carry out your wishes. In the midst of conflicting advice, well-meaning help that is sometimes more of a hindrance, undermining comments and judgements from those around you, the doula may well be the one person who says things like: 'How does that feel? You're doing so well. How do you feel your baby is doing? What would you like to do? What do you think you need?'

Like other mammals, we learn by example. We are a circle of mothers, evolved as a tribal species. Without our womenfolk around us, passing on the wisdom and practical skills, is it any wonder that breastfeeding has become mysterious and difficult and oh, so lonely?

> *After listening to a client for ages the thing she kept repeating was "and the poor dog isn't getting walked", so I did that and by the time I got back babe was happily feeding – funny that!*
>
> Debra Virchis

We see you bring her to the breast. We smile encouragingly. Remind you to keep her close, so close no one can see where your body ends and hers begins. She feels safe, part of you, as her belly and chest sink into you. She feels her chin planted squarely on your warm, sweet-smelling breast. She reaches up, tipping her heavy head back, gaping open with her hot mouth and you draw her ever closer. Her search is over. Her whole body melts as the warm, sweet milk begins to flow.

Whether you choose to breastfeed, formula feed or a bit of both, whether you are determined to reach your goals, or intend to go with the flow, you are not feeding your baby in isolation. You are the product of millions of years of history and culture and subject to the whims and pressures of this particular point in history.

Today we use breasts to sell cars and newspapers, we enlarge them, lift them, encase them in lace and show them off (as long as no areola or nipple peeps out, of course!). They are simultaneously our badge of womanhood and our cross to bear. We are judged and judge ourselves on the state of our jugs and simultaneously worry that they may let us down, sag, lose their allure or even kill us. Somewhere along the line we've forgotten what these mammary glands are for. It seems our culture has swallowed the misguided notion that breasts are genitalia. And if that is the case, how on earth do we get them out of our bras and attach babies to them?

If, like me, you have worried all your life about how your body is seen by others, defining your self-worth by your size and shape, breastfeeding can seem particularly complex. Are these second-rate tits up to the job? Are they fit for public consumption? We are taught that our bodies are fragile and liable to break down. We constantly compare ourselves to the most beautiful and find ourselves wanting.

Those of us who work in this world of breasts and bodies have to inhabit a shadowy world of taboo, hang-ups, revulsion and longing. People have complicated relationships with their bodies. We have to explore the hinterlands of our own attitudes; understanding that the way we fed our babies and how we feel are all irrelevant: this is all about *you*.

The social mores of our time are that mothers are expected to breastfeed. We are encouraged to at least give it a go. Everyone bangs on about the benefits to the baby. Many of us assume breastfeeding is a natural instinct: how hard can it be? Hardly anyone talks about the potential dark side of breastfeeding – the challenges and the pain – in case mothers are put off.

The result? Mothers who are inadequately prepared and who lack good support. The irony is that if mothers don't know about the possible challenges they may encounter, they are more likely to encounter them, more likely to assume they are normal or that nothing can be done about them, and less likely to seek help. It's like trying to learn survival skills, in the jungle, alone, armed only with a butter knife.

Because… here's the thing: breastfeeding is driven by an engine of instincts, hormones and reflexes in both you and your baby. You may need a little bit of help to learn to control that engine. Knowing when to change gear, accelerate and break, judging your speed, the needs and intentions of your fellow road users and gaining confidence as a driver is a subtle process of learning and growth. But, like driving, nursing soon becomes a thoughtless action, one that can be done while having a conversation and thinking about what you're going to cook for your evening meal.

But without someone to sit next to you in the passenger seat, what happens? Mothers can feel betrayed, let down and pressurised… or maybe, even more sadly, think they have failed and are riddled with guilt. The reality is that they have been failed by the very system that was meant to support them. And these mothers can feel bitter. Some will even spread the idea that breastfeeding is painful and difficult and lots of people just can't do it. This isn't really true. And it doesn't do much to help *you* achieve *your* goals, in your way, with your baby.

So many women get so little skilled support in the early days that lots of women out there are either learning to drive all by themselves, or being guided by people who are passing on misunderstandings, myths and over-generalisations. That means there are lots of people crunching their gears, or even stalling the car altogether. Some people might imply that if you just *try* a little harder, or wait a little longer, it will all work out. Some might try to tell you it's your fault you're finding it difficult. Of course that won't help if you never know not to crunch those gears or if your baby has challenges of her own. It means that sore nipples or achy breasts or other worries don't get addressed. Just because something is common, doesn't make it normal.

There are lots of reasons why we've got to this place; not least through the influence of the powerful multinationals that have a vested interest in your baby not breastfeeding. Along the way, culture, economics and big business have taught us not to trust our bodies.

From conception to birth to feeding our babies, technology and capitalism pave our way and cushion us from the visceral experience of our mammalian nature. It appears that the more disconnected we are from our bodies, the more we rely on science, money and technology, even believing it to be superior to the model that nearly two million years of evolution has perfected. The bottle has become the symbol of motherhood – the iconography is everywhere: on baby-changing rooms, congratulations cards and in the media.

Our bodies have become a necessary evil – we leak unsavoury fluids and are inconvenienced by pain and dysfunction. And from unsavoury and inconvenient, it's only one small step to distasteful, abhorrent and eventually, taboo. These complicated feelings and powerful cultural messages can have a real and tangible effect on your experience of motherhood.

The last couple of generations have seen a resurgence in interest in breastfeeding. But there's a good chance your mother and even your grandmother bottle-fed their children. Women are growing up disconnected from nursing, without the faintest clue how a baby latches or the natural rhythms of a nursing newborn.

When our mothers had babies, it was believed that formula was a modern, scientific advance on nature. In the age of female emancipation, the bottle offered a freedom that ordinary women, without access to wet nurses, had never had. The idea that breastfeeding, and therefore being somehow 'chained' to the baby, is a rather anti-feminist pursuit is still prevalent. But the notion that a woman must resist the temptation to give in to her biological urges to make love, procreate and lactate in order to earn her feminist stripes is, of course, nonsense.

It is only in recent years that we have begun to gain a deeper understanding of the way that breastfeeding works. What I mean is that we have had a very simplistic notion of how to teach a mother to breastfeed – that it is she who is the 'doer' and the baby the 'receiver'.

We have been sold an idea of breastfeeding as a series of ritualised movements or steps that are the same for everyone. A very 'mother-led' activity, measured out by the clock into arbitrary slices of time. Actually, it is the baby who breastfeeds – the mother merely provides the habitat (her body), her attention and her desire to nurse. Provided that you and your baby are allowed to bathe in an oxytocin-rich environment, the chances are that your baby will latch, and keep latching.

When you look up from your bubble to ask if things are 'right' or 'normal', your doula will give you the same kind of support that she would provide in labour – reassurance, and quiet faith in your ability to know your body and your baby. 'How does it feel?' 'Is your baby enjoying it?' 'You know how to do this – the knowing is deep inside both of you'.

Sadly, much of what we do during birth and immediately after serves to impede this oxytocin-rich environment post-birth. Drugs and instruments and surgical procedures can put a brake on the baby's natural reflexes to find the breast. Even after a drug-free birth, little things can burst the oxytocin bubble:

- The baby having a very 'hands-on delivery' so she may feel tense or experience discomfort.
- Early cord-clamping, which can interrupt the 'birth pause' and speed up and disrupt the baby's transition from womb to world.
- Separation of mother and baby – delaying skin-to-skin and potentially missing that golden window when everything maximises the possibility of the baby latching without hindrance.
- Baby cleaned and wrapped; disrupting those magical moments of smell and touch as the baby finds her own way to the breast.

- The baby being presented to the mother; laid in her arms rather than in chest-to-chest contact. I have noticed that rather than the instinctive discovering of each other that happens naturally when mother and baby are chest-to-chest – the mother shifting slightly and making her body available to her wriggling infant – when the baby is lying on her back in the mother's arms, the mother is more likely to look up and ask what she needs to do to 'feed the baby'.
- All the other fuss of a standard delivery unit and excited family members – hats, weighing, vitamin K injections, the hurrying of the third stage, bright lights, staff coming and going, phone calls made, photos taken.
- The mother or baby being washed too soon. The smell imprinting necessary for safe attachment is well understood in animals, but rarely discussed in humans.
- The mother not kept totally warm, thus lowering her oxytocin levels, possibly delaying the birth of the placenta and making it less likely that the environment will be primed for the baby self-attaching.
- The mother not feeling safe, private and unobserved. This affects her oxytocin levels.
- The 'baby-to-boob head shove'. This 'technique', which involves grabbing the mother's breast and the baby's head and pushing the two together in the hope they will stick has, in my experience, caused more anguish than almost any other routine postnatal procedure. Mothers complain of feeling bruised, violated and alarmed by the violence of the gesture. Babies make their feelings known as well – by refusing to latch, screaming every time they see a breast, arching back against that strong hand on the back of her head. If someone rudely pushed on the back of your head, what would you want to do?

I humbly suggest not letting anyone do that to your precious baby. Like any jigsaw puzzle, it doesn't help to force the pieces together.

The desire to have a baby is imprinted deep in our genetic coding. It is not a rational, neo-cortical decision. Likewise, the inclination to the put the baby to the breast is a biological urge. It is a feeling, deep in our wombs and hearts and guts. When our babies flail around and don't latch; when they push against us and arch away; when they spit out the nipple; when this thing we yearn to do *hurts*; when our nipples bleed or when our beloved babies don't gain weight; when all around us talk about the ease and advantages of formula; when lactation seems just too hard to master, the grief can be deep and damaging. The sense of rejection and failure can be all-consuming and the anger can be debilitating.

The combination of massive formula company marketing budgets, low-quality training for health professionals, zero understanding of how breastfeeding works among the general population and the deep hurt of some mothers has resulted in a culture of fear and distrust of breastfeeding. When pain and regret collides with the understandable pride and joyful flush of oxytocin that bathes breastfeeding mothers, sparks can fly. How convenient for the formula companies, as they portray themselves as the supporters of mothers who are victims of the 'mummy wars'. In any discourse a minority are evangelical and judgemental, on all sides of every debate. In general though, if you are breastfeeding and someone tuts, they are just a product of their culture. If you are formula-feeding and a mother talks about how happy she is to be breastfeeding, she isn't trying to make you feel guilty – she's just enjoying her choice and expressing her pride. Be happy for her.

You might be reading this and wondering why so many

people get their knickers in a twist about infant feeding. We are surrounded by outwardly healthy gorgeous children who were formula-fed. We are lucky, in the West, to have access to electricity, clean water and high-quality health care. However, the fact remains that at a population level, even in developed countries, formula feeding affects the health of mothers and babies. Formula is lacking in many of the properties that are necessary for optimal health and development. That is no one's fault – we just can't reproduce a living, ever-changing fluid in a factory.

Formula can be contaminated. It boringly tastes the same, every single meal. Air miles, landfill rubbish and the use of water and electricity contribute to the global ecological disaster that threatens to engulf us. The companies that sell it use unethical marketing practices, break laws and violate an international code designed by the World Health Organisation to protect all mothers – those who are breastfeeding and those who use formula. The companies are trying very hard to get to *you*. They market other products with similar branding, persuade health professionals to endorse their products and spend millions on advertising. The costs of marketing are passed on to the parents – if formula advertising was controlled in the way that campaigners are pushing for, formula could be available at a fraction of its current retail price.

Formula saves lives. When there is a clear medical need, we are lucky to have access to a milk food that will usually ensure our babies' safety. If, for whatever reason, breastfeeding isn't for you, you deserve access to unbiased, evidence-based information about formula together with non-judgemental support to feed your baby in a way that suits you both. You certainly deserve an affordable, high-quality product that is well regulated, comprising ingredients that experts agree are optimal and safe.

Mothers have the right to purchase a product that is

presented in packaging that doesn't lead them to believe, through health claims and strap lines, that this product will be better for their babies than the competition. Babies are far too important for expensive formulas to be better for your baby than cheaper brands. No food regulatory agency would allow that. They are all the same, so choose one that seems to suit your baby and that you can afford and get hold of easily.

Normal newborns feed *at least* 8 to 14 times in 24 hours. Often they feed almost constantly in the evenings! Sometimes, when they are very little, it's hard to know when one 'feed' ends and another begins. But there will be respite – they do sleep sometimes. Part of the reason nature set it up this way is to make you sit, rest, nurse, recover from childbirth, stare at your baby and be tended to. If you haven't got someone fanning you with a palm frond and peeling you grapes, consider reaching out to friends, family or your doula.

There are many and varied discussions about things like the size of newborns' stomachs, the rate at which milk is digested, the newborn's need for sleep in order to grow and the baby's need to suckle for reasons other than purely nutritional. It might help to understand that breasts are factories, not warehouses; you are never empty. And when you feel, at the end of the day, that your factory really must have gone on strike, your milk, while low in volume, is super fatty and comforting – an evening cocoa for a baby who has been working hard all day getting used to the world.

We all have a unique 'storage capacity'; in other words, the volume of milk we can store in our boobs at any one time. A woman with a large storage capacity may fill her baby up to the brim and find her baby tends to feed less often. Those of us with smaller capacities may have a baby who needs to suckle more frequently. The amount of milk each mother makes in a whole day, however, may be pretty much the same and capacity is not connected to the size of your boobs.

Like any factory, if the customer is asking for more, the workforce has to ramp up production. If you feed less, perhaps because you are using some bottles, the factory will compensate by slowing down production. In this way, our body and baby work together to make sure we make enough milk for our babies, but not too much, which would be uncomfortable. The system works well for most dyads, but not so well for a few, so if you feel you have too much or too little milk, get some skilled support.

Because you can expect your newborn to want to hang out on or near your breast pretty much constantly, Mother Nature has set up a system of rewards: the hormones of breastfeeding are feel-good relaxants, reducing stress and sometimes sending you off into a rather blissed-out state. Mother Nature *wants* you to breastfeed, not for days or weeks, or months, but years. So she makes it a rewarding experience. If your nipples hurt, or anything else is upsetting you about your breastfeeding, this is not what the system intended – and there is an army of skilled, passionate women out there, aching to help you... and keep on helping you until everything is fine, or you tell them to clear off.

Babies are hardwired to have physical contact with another human body and to suckle frequently. Babies suckle for food, drink, pain relief, reassurance, to go to sleep, to wake up, for entertainment and for other emotions any human being might experience. We have spent the last couple of hundred years trying to deny that humans are a carrying species, earnestly trying to get mothers to feed and comfort their babies by the clock and transport them with wheels. Fortunately, babies (or your breasts!) can't tell the time – nor can they usually be fooled by vibrating chairs or expensive prams. They may tolerate them, but what your baby really needs in the early days is you. You may like to explore the idea of a sling/cloth carrier – babies have evolved to expect to be carried, but grown-ups need their hands free. A sling keeps both parties happy.

Babies are just small humans, and most adults enjoy oral and skin-to-skin stimulation. We eat, drink, kiss, cuddle and some of us smoke. The needs we have as babies continue throughout life.

There really are only three rules to breastfeeding: 1. Feed the baby (by hook or by crook, in whatever manner and with whatever milk – yours, another woman's or modified from a cow – your baby will need feeding). 2. Protect your milk supply (if you take out your milk, by putting your baby to the breast, or expressing with your hand, or pumping with a machine, you will send a strong signal to your brain to make milk. If you make milk, you can fulfil Rule 1. 3. Keep your baby close (if you have close contact, including skin-to-skin, you will stimulate your supply and fulfil Rule 2, and encourage your baby to latch frequently, which fulfils Rule 1 and Rule 2).

If your nipples are comfy, your baby is weeing and pooing, has some settled times and she's getting bigger, you can probably rest assured that things are going swimmingly. If not, or you have any anxieties, pick up the phone or go to a support group. There will be someone, somewhere who has the key to unlock the door to pleasurable breastfeeding. Most of them, trained by the charitable breastfeeding organisations, should support you free of charge.

Your doula will be your signpost, pointing you towards skilled, loving, knowledgeable, non-judgemental breastfeeding supporters. The groups they run are a safe haven, even if you don't have any challenges to overcome. The friendships mothers make in these groups can last a lifetime.

Helping mothers learn to breastfeed their babies is the most satisfying work in the world; I've never found anything that's so much worth doing. Rachel O'Leary, IBCLC

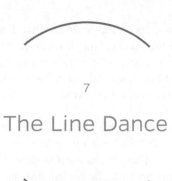

7

The Line Dance

The elderly lady bends painfully and peers into the pram, cooing. After a few moments praising her blue eyes and double chin, she straightens up, looks at my client and asks 'Is she a good baby? Does she sleep through yet?' I notice my client's white knuckles on the pram handle. I glance at her set jaw and tired eyes. There is a pause.

I smile across at the woman and say gently, 'Aren't all babies good? She's a blessing'. She grins, and nods and we all go on our way. My client chatters on the way home, but once we are ensconced in the kitchen with a cup of tea, she bursts into tears. She is full of fear and doubt and concern. What if her baby is broken? What if she's a terrible mother? Is there something she should be doing, to tame and train her baby?

Many of my clients are being told that babies are creatures to be tamed. If one doesn't train a baby like a puppy, break its spirit and show it who's pack leader, it will grow up to be a chaotic nuisance, gnawing on the furniture and leaving puddles on the laminate.

It's only since becoming a doula that I've realised how polarised parenting has become. It seems that the overarching social attitudes, at least here in Britain, are that children should be seen and not heard, should not impact on the mother's life and are a serious threat to her sexual and economic availability.

> *I remember saying to [my friend], 'Look, Amelie's crying – what do I do? Pick her up or leave her there?' She gently replied 'What do you want to do?' 'Pick her up!' I said. 'Pick her up then,' she smiled. This was the biggest lesson of parenting for me.*
>
> Lisa Ramsey

In modern society, getting to grips with parenthood can be tough. Isolation, the economic realities of work outside the home and a never-ending stream of conflicting advice from friends, family and the internet can be rather overwhelming. The choices and soul-searching we increasingly do in pregnancy about the way we wish to birth, don't end in the birth room. In fact, one of the reasons I encourage parents to start making choices in pregnancy is because this choosing, planning and organising is not going to stop – for at least eighteen years! From where your baby sleeps to what college to choose, your life will be measured out in decisions. Getting into the habit of looking at all sides of a question and taking the option that suits you best may well stand you in good stead as the years roll by.

As your child grows, so you will blossom as a parent. What often seems to help is when parents find their tribe; friends and family who will cheer their successes and commiserate when things are tough. Many of us have been disconnected from a social support network that can nurture and sustain us through the joys and challenges of the early years of parenting.

This is partly because, in a world where a large proportion of mothers are going back to full-time work, we have a limited window of time in which to make friendships that will sustain us. This is one reason why antenatal classes, postnatal groups, and breastfeeding support groups are so crucial. Groups need to be facilitated by sensitive, knowledgeable people, so that facts can be shared instead of horror stories and everyone is welcomed without judgement.

Groups also need to be able to welcome the whole family; mothers, fathers, older siblings, grandparents. Separating mothers and babies from their families, or their supporters from their children, seems short-sighted to me. Once women would have been surrounded by their female tribe: friends, neighbours, family. Older women to pass on the wisdom and to look up to, younger women looking up to us, girls jostling with each other to hold a baby, or play with the toddler. We were never alone in our doubt and guilt and worry and always had someone to share the joy and the pride in our achievements. It wouldn't have been perfect, of course: judgement and gossip and nosiness aren't modern inventions. These days we have access to unprecedented amounts of information, good housing, sanitation and health care. But something is definitely missing. I see an almost tangible gaping abyss at the heart of many new mothers. They yearn for something they don't even know they are missing.

Modern parents are all too often alone and lonely. It's not that we can't do it by ourselves, it's just that it's hard, and not as much fun. We didn't evolve to do this job alone. So if you struggle, it is not your fault. If you wobble and worry, it's not your fault. If your dreams are dashed and regret casts a shadow over your days, it is not your fault. And you are definitely not alone.

The line dance of raising a child is a long, tiring and exhilarating one. Sometimes, when the music is quiet, there dances the mother alone, with her baby in her arms. At other times, there are many dancers; sometimes, few. Sometimes mother or father sits out, watching the dance and resting. Sometimes everyone joins in and exalts in the rousing music. Always the dancers move to the same tune; the music and the pace always set by the parents, their steps gently guided by the more experienced dancers. The steps of the dance are simple, the rhythm comes naturally when the dancers just follow the beat. Sometimes new dancers stumble, yet there is always someone there to steady them again. When the music is jolly, we watch you dance with joy in our hearts. When the melody is sad or stormy, we move in to accompany you and shield you from harm.

Find your tribe, your fellow dancers, and parenting can be a whole lot easier, more fun and less anxious. The phrase I hear uttered most often when I take a client to a mother's group or breastfeeding support clinic is, 'Oh, it's not just me, then?' No. No it's not.

One of my greatest pleasures as a doula is when I help a mum find her tribe. It might be introducing her to another client who lives nearby, or taking her to a mother support group or even, these days, pointing her towards a support group on social media. Some of my clients have joined forces and set up a local VBAC support group. It's what I mean when I tell my doula trainees that doulas are 'social glue'.

When you feel that you belong, when you feel truly heard, you feel strong and capable of being the mother or father you want to be.

Separation from our tribe can have far-reaching consequences. It is no coincidence that high rates of postnatal depression are associated with communities that have low levels of social integration and where mothers suffer isolation and a lack of support. This exclusion from social support structures is a problem that affects everyone – some of my most lonely, anxious clients have been those living in the biggest houses, in the most affluent areas of town.

Where there is isolation, there follows a greater risk of domestic violence, self-harm or neglect. On average two women a week are killed by a male partner or former partner. A third of domestic violence starts in pregnancy and has been identified as a leading cause of miscarriage and stillbirth. Higher rates of violence against women are found where women's status is lowest; where there are clear inequalities between men and women, rigid gender roles and cultural norms that support a man's 'right' to sex.

How we view women, and mothers in particular, is more than just an academic or political argument. If women and children are to be kept safe and healthy, social support and the status of women is crucial.

Since women became divorced from our traditional female support structures, we have begun to lean more heavily on our menfolk in the time around childbirth. An enormous shift has occurred in only one generation. When I was born in 1969, my father dropped my mother at the front door of the hospital and went to work. He didn't reappear until I was a few hours old. He never spoke of how he felt about leaving her, but my mother has a vivid memory of holding onto a young student midwife's hand for dear life as she pushed. I like to think my country-boy Dad was at work, unconcerned in his faith that females just have babies. I hope so. Because what I see more often these days are fathers who are petrified, or at least very unsure of their role. From banishing men entirely, in the space of 40 years we have turned things around so spectacularly that now, if a couple prefer for him not to be at the birth, or if he expresses reservations or fears, he is judged and shamed.

When we took birth out of the home in the 1960s and 70s and removed women from their traditional support structures, we felt the emotional and spiritual emptiness of hospital birth. For many, hospital was a place of illness and death, full of strangers and frightening machines, bright lights and unintelligible jargon. No wonder we wanted a loved one there, someone who made us feel safe. As doctors took more control of childbirth, and most of them were men, perhaps women thought bringing their own man might even up the balance a little! Many fathers have stepped up to the role of birth companion with aplomb. Loving, sensitive, tireless in their physical and emotional support: some men have a natural gift for this work. I know a couple of wonderful male midwives who prove that gender is no barrier to effective care in pregnancy and childbirth.

> *Sam was the best male doula (moula?) I could have ever hoped for and the best dad from word go. I have never felt more supported and in partnership [with him] than throughout the wait for both my very overdue children or throughout their very different births. His trust and belief in me were greater than my own and he has never said anything except positive comments about the experience or about my strength. Awesome example of alpha stepping aside for goddess.*
>
> Kay King

Many men, however, are filled with adrenaline as soon as contractions begin. Those 3 'f's can take their toll, with them either getting grumpy and aggressive (fight), looking a little like a rabbit in the headlights (freeze), or disappearing on some small errand for hours (flight). I have seen all of these responses and a few more, including the compulsive need to make jokes, and a couple of guys who passed out (that would be the fourth f – faint!).

I have also come to believe that no one has an automatic

right to be present during labour and birth. It is the woman doing this incredible job. She is the queen bee and she calls the shots about who graces her with their presence. That goes for everyone – family, staff or doulas.

We have not responded as a culture to men in the birth room with any great effectiveness. Antenatal education classes do their best to show partners how they can best support their women during birth and through the babymoon, but the provision varies greatly around the country.

When I work with a couple, I try hard to get across the message that, in fact, the partner has a crucial part to play. His feelings about his role, and what she wants and needs from him, are important to share. If they are a loving couple, the oxytocin they can produce together, as they gaze into each other's eyes, kiss, cuddle and touch, is more powerful than any artificial hormone drip. He can be home, safety, privacy, labour progression, lover, advocate and protector all rolled into one. But he doesn't always have to be by her side to give her exactly what she needs.

In a hospital delivery room a father looked at me, concern and confusion in his eyes. Shoulders hunched, I could see the adrenaline coursing through his veins. I smiled. I motioned with my eyes to come closer and encouraged him to lay his hand on his wife's shoulder and whisper sweet nothings in her ear. She was nearing full dilation, the contractions rocking her with their intensity. With his warm hand on her skin and the sound of his voice in her ear she visibly relaxed. Soon she was pushing and the atmosphere in the room lightened. He looked at me again and grinned.

For a woman, having her significant other there with her on this amazing day can be incredible. The love and connection that put the baby in there, can really help to get the baby out. But equally, I've known fathers who do not wish to be there, or at least not in an active role. I've met women who love their partner dearly, but laugh at the idea of having him present, or know that it will be beyond his capabilities to support her in the way she needs. There is no judgement in that knowledge; why should there be? You may encounter people who have strong opinions about men in the birthing room. I think it's time we moved away from old-fashioned notions of gender. Instead we should ask: 'Will this person bring oxytocin or adrenaline into the room?' and 'What do the parents want?'

During my years of doulaing I've met many fathers. Often, it is the father who wants the doula. Sometimes it's even the father who makes the initial call. The myth that doulas are only there for the mother and can even have a negative impact on the ability of the father to support his wife persists. But it isn't what I see.

Take the father who remembered trying to support his wife first time round in the hospital. He had no idea how best to comfort and support her, and they had been left alone for long periods of time in the busy delivery unit. No one offered him drinks or snacks and he didn't feel he could leave his wife. Frankly, he'd been terrified and, after a long labour and birth, was faint with hunger and dehydration. This time, he wanted a help-mate and companion. I tended to them both when she went into labour. I fed and watered them, fetched and carried, made the tea, showed him how to massage her back, to dance with her during contractions, to love and care for her through each surge until the baby made his entrance.

I remember the father who was very, very squeamish – he feared fainting at the sight of his girlfriend losing blood, vomiting or, his worst fear, pushing out the baby. He was so worried that he would be expected to watch and cut the cord. During the time we spent together antenatally, they decided to stay at home for the birth. This way he could come and go as he pleased, within his comfort zone. He managed to be in the room when the baby was born and was very proud of himself.

I have also met more than one man suffering from a birth trauma that he has never been allowed to express. The memory of nearly losing a loved one, or not knowing what is happening, can have an enormous ripple effect across a couple's childbearing years – and even affect their marriage.

Doulas work alongside many grandmothers and a few grandfathers. I have shared birth spaces with some grandmothers who were wonderful supports to their daughters. I have also run up and down corridors to waiting rooms to convey news of the progress of labour to anxious waiting relatives. Sometimes the doula is the glue that sticks a family together.

Of course, it is often the woman who wants the doula. It's not uncommon for the father to not really understand why. Usually they just want their partner to be happy and comfortable, so will happily welcome the doula into the birth space. It's my job to make sure his fears and anxieties are addressed and that he feels supported too. Here's how one father felt about having a doula:

> *Throughout the labour... our doula's experience and quiet reassurance kept us both focused... calm and relaxed. At no point did we become fearful. Her balance was perfect – whether just being observational, or providing support – we felt that she was able to ensure that we followed our preferences and create the ideal environment. Importantly she also ensured that the midwife was aligned to our preferences. Once we had the most beautiful girl, we did have to transfer into hospital unfortunately due to a retained placenta. Our doula supported us throughout the time spent waiting for the procedure in hospital, and did not leave until she was*

satisfied that we were all OK in recovery. At a time when we were all very emotional and tired, she was again a calming and reassuring influence.

Simon Graham

It can sometimes be a challenge for a father to understand his wife's preferences and choices. Why would she dream of a normal birth after the frightening labour and emergency c-section last time? Why would she risk planning to stay at home to have the baby? Why does she want to invite this strange woman on our private journey? Isn't formula feeding a simpler, more controlled and measurable way to feed the baby, that will enable him to help her?

Inviting a doula to participate in these discussions can help facilitate effective communication, and allow mutual understanding to grow and concerns to be put into context. A doula may provide the father with evidence-based reading material or suggest a health professional to talk to so that he understands the risks and benefits of his partner's choices. The result is a birth 'dream-team' – two sets of hands to support her, two loving companions to hold her birth space and have faith in her ability to birth this baby beautifully.

I have been invited to share the journey by families who have no available friends or family close by to care for older children while the parents get on with the business of birthing. At a home birth, there's often more than enough work for two – inflating and filling the birth pool, answering the phone or greeting the midwives at the door. Making snacks, topping up the warm water in the pool, fetching and carrying are all part of the doula remit. As one of the fathers I once supported said:

It was such a relief to me when you arrived, as you helped take the pressure off me... I was tired, and trying to be so supportive to her for so long was mentally exhausting.

Of course, the birth is only the beginning. As the mother's supreme efforts finish, the 24/7 work of caring for the baby begins. Doula care naturally flows into this space too. This morning, I made breakfast, held the baby while the mother had a bath, did the washing-up, chatted about breastfeeding and kept the mother company while the father got some much-needed work done. In a quiet moment, I talked to them both about the amazing capabilities of their newborn, helping them recognise her sophisticated attempts at communication. I left the parents cooing over their newborn, caressing the soft hair on her head.

As doula means 'servant', it is always with that in mind that I serve the family – adapting to their ever-changing needs and mindful that families need fathers who are happy, strong, capable and confident in their parenting. And of course, I'm not forgetting all the other flavours of families I have worked for. However many parents there are, and whatever their genders, they all need support to find their feet as parents and to build a loving home for their children.

As a doula, a feminist and a human being, I believe I am here to listen to what everyone is saying. As a passionate advocate of choice, how can I not hear a man when he expresses his preferences, and how can I not work to create an environment where he can be what he needs to be and do what he needs to do? I am continually amazed at how couples manage to find a way to meet both their differing sets of needs. Compromise and necessity are the parents of invention!

We live in a culture which is slowly becoming aware that fathers are under greater social and economic pressure than ever. It is known that they suffer from birth trauma and postnatal depression too. In that context, the need for social support is greater than ever. I don't care whether it's a doula, sister, in-laws or the lady next door who provides it, as long as they get it.

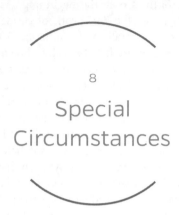

8

Special Circumstances

We are lucky to live in a country where, despite all the much-needed improvements in maternity care, birth is generally safe. The vast majority of mothers and babies come out physically unscathed. Most women in Western countries embark on their first pregnancy assuming that all will be well, especially after reaching that all-important first scan date.

Not all of us, however, can look back on an ecstatic birth or a joyful babymoon. Some of us will have to experience the rollercoaster of emotions that accompany a child in special care, while others will come out the other side of childbirth shell-shocked, like a soldier emerging from the trenches. Some will find that parenthood throws up emotional challenges that take them to a very dark place indeed, while others have to grapple with the greatest grief of all; the loss of a child.

More commonly, women end up giving birth in a way that they hadn't planned, or make choices that have repercussions they didn't expect. This chapter can do little more than scratch the surface of some of these topics, but I hope to show that doulas can make an enormous difference when parents are facing challenges, tough choices or walking their dark night of the soul.

Freebirth

Some might wonder why freebirth is included in this chapter – it is not a 'challenge' or a 'problem' – while others may criticise me for including it at all, for fear of encouraging women to birth alone. However, freebirth is a subject us doulas are obliged to grapple with, so it must be included here. The fact is, sometimes women choose to birth alone. This choice takes many forms and may be motivated by many things.

The definition of unassisted childbirth, or freebirth, is fluid. Sometimes women feel they have no choice other than to disengage from maternity services. This may be because they have lost trust in their midwives or doctors. It is sometimes because their informed choices and birth wishes are being blocked at every turn. Others have experienced sexual or other kinds of controlling abuse in their past and feel unable to engage with a service that at times can feel controlling and very powerful. Increasingly, mothers are so traumatised by a previous birth experience, that they cannot imagine being in that same environment again or meeting any of the staff involved. Like any major trauma, many things can trigger renewed suffering, flashbacks and debilitating fear or other strong emotions. To avoid this, sometimes women withdraw themselves, partially or completely, from the system.

Not all freebirthing comes from a negative perspective. For some, the innate knowledge that their bodies work most efficiently and safely in complete privacy, uninhibited by the presence of anyone, other than their immediate family, leads them to choose this path. As Vicki Williams, freebirthing mother, says:

There is a big misconception that if the maternity services

> *got it right women would stop freebirthing, but I don't think that is the case. Some would, but the majority of those who seek the privacy and intimacy that freebirth offers would no more invite a midwife to join them at the birth than at the conception – even those who count some very good midwives among their close personal friends.*

Many believe that freebirthing is illegal. Some people even mistakenly believe that birthing alone, whether deliberately or accidentally, is against the law and only health professionals can catch babies. No father has ever been criminalised for catching his own hastily-born child. Nor has a woman been prosecuted for planning a freebirth. The law is clear: a woman has the unalienable right to birth where, and with whoever, she chooses. It is not illegal to catch a baby. It is, however, illegal to masquerade as a health professional. In other words, it would be just as bad to dress up as a midwife and go around catching babies as it would to strut around the hospital with a stethoscope around your neck pretending to be a doctor. This kind of behaviour would be reprehensible; people need to know they can trust their public servants. But if your partner or your doula ends up helping you catch your baby, no law has been broken, as long as no one misled you about their qualifications and clinical role.

Beyond misunderstandings of the law, freebirthing often attracts judgement and astonishment. The public and many health professionals find it hard to understand why a mother might make this choice. As a doula, I have been appalled at the way these women can be treated. The negative reaction they may get if they admit to a midwife that they may choose to go without medical support in labour generally only serves to entrench that mother even more firmly in her freebirthing plans. I have found that really listening to her, making no judgement of her choice, validating her feelings and helping her explore all the possibilities open to her is a much more loving approach and without doubt provides a safer environment for that mother – whatever she ultimately decides to do.

I am well aware that some 'whoops' births are unconscious freebirths; the mother has been unable to admit to herself or to anyone else that she doesn't want to call a midwife or go to hospital. It's amazing what our subconscious can achieve for us sometimes when our primal instincts are in direct opposition to our higher, thinking brain. I have been with women who are clearly struggling to work out, between intense contractions, what it is they feel they need. I always tell them during pregnancy that, in labour, they will 'just know 'where their safe birth nest is, who they need to be there and when they need to go there. When a woman looks at me and asks, 'Is it time to call the midwife?' I tend to say, 'If you're asking me that, then yes'.

Despite the incredible pressures that maternity services are under at this point in history, despite the spectacular difficulties midwives encounter every day trying to provide a safe, holistic, loving service, despite the fear and trauma and the lack of safe places to deal with those feelings, they manage to step up, often. I believe and know that they can, and often do, bend over backwards to give a woman what she needs, however unusual. Supervisors of midwives can be angels from heaven. A consultant midwife sometimes knows the magic word that will open many doors and make possible many choices. Personally, politically, I am a believer in the NHS and I want to give them the chance to show how awesome they are. I, and my clients, have had a few knocks over the years, but like any believer it takes a lot to undermine my faith.

Great, even spectacular, care is out there but not all women are treated gently and intelligently when it comes to freebirth. I would never persuade a woman to re-engage with a service that she feels is dangerous for her or undermining of her informed decisions. Sometimes there is a clear and present danger for women in this situation; AIMS has a list of cases of women who have been coerced, harassed or even reported to social services for their freebirthing choices.

As doulas, freebirthing is both a simple and a very complex subject. Some in our community have freebirthed themselves and are happy to consider an invitation to be present in a house while a freebirth is happening. This may be to care for older children or to tend to the parents' practical needs while they labour together. Every doula must go on her own process of reflection if she is asked to accompany a mother on her freebirthing journey. It is not just a decision about the concept of freebirth itself, but a deep reflection on what the mother needs and whether this doula can work with this mother in a spirit of mutual love and trust.

While doulas have no clinical responsibility for the outcome and no legal responsibility for the safety of the mother or baby, it is a personal decision whether a doula would feel a moral responsibility. Would I call 999 against the parents' wishes if something dreadful occurred? Would I recognise the signs of things going wrong? Would I shoulder the burden of that moral responsibility, even if the parents don't want me to? If the worst happened, would I torture myself with the what-ifs for ever? What if something dreadful happened and the world, or the parents, blamed the doula? Although we do not provide a medical birth support service, we do provide a birth support service and sometimes get paid for that. It can be hard for the public, and sometimes the police, to work out what that means and to feel reassured a doula hasn't crossed her boundaries. This is deep, dark, complicated stuff and it is not for me to dictate what any mother or her doula chooses to do.

Our membership organisation, Doula UK, has grappled

with this subject. Our code of conduct, updated in 2014, reiterates the legal right of a mother to birth as she chooses, but stresses that the organisation isn't a union and cannot provide legal representation or financial help for a doula accused of crossing her boundaries by going to a freebirth.

Birth trauma

The first time I saw Jane after having her second baby, I didn't recognise her. Without red-rimmed eyes and drooping shoulders, she looked younger and those eyes were softened and devoid of pain. When I'd first met her, she rarely did anything other than weep. The story of her first birth played on a loop in her mind, day and night. She found it hard to eat.

Many doulas find themselves supporting women with birth trauma. We might be the birth doula, helping a woman approach a subsequent birth and deal with the fears a new pregnancy brings, or perhaps the postnatal doula supporting her through the fall-out of a traumatic birth. I also meet women through my breastfeeding support role who are struggling with much more than feeding their babies.

A woman's journey through birth trauma will be her story to tell. What helps and hinders is unique to each mother. Sometimes, making an official complaint about the care she received will be cathartic. Other mothers may benefit from specialist therapies and counselling, and some might just need a friend, relative or doula to support her through the tough times. Others will bury the memory and focus their energies on the baby. Many feel healed after a subsequent well-supported birth.

Disappointment in life (and in birth) is inevitable. If you are dealing with the disappointment of a birth not going to plan, remember that it is always okay to feel sad. You might feel very sad indeed and feel a need to grieve deeply for what you didn't have. That's okay. But never blame yourself. Never feel that you should have done something differently. Or said something else. Or planned for it differently. For this is unkind and unfair on you. And not realistic. Birth is not like running a marathon. It is more like recovering from flu. Sometimes it goes well and sometimes it doesn't. But you can't control the outcome. And it's not your fault. So seek the support of others and acknowledge your need to grieve as well as to celebrate the birth of your baby. It may seem odd but it is possible to feel happy and sad at the same time.

If you find that you can't feel happy at all because the birth is too upsetting, don't keep this to yourself. Get some help from family, your GP, your friends, health visitor or midwife. Or even better, your doula.

Mia Scotland, clinical psychologist and antenatal teacher

Trauma comes in many guises and is caused by any number of situations. Trauma is not in the eye of the beholder; what would be experienced as a nightmare by one woman might be dismissed as trivial by another. One experience is not 'worse' than others. We do not get to judge a woman's right to feel traumatised. Her birth story belongs to her. Her emotions belong to her. Sometimes, childbirth reignites old trauma or triggers deep wounds. Our role is to accept her pain and hold the space for her while she works out what she needs on her journey to a place of peace.

We met our doula, Lisa, when she did a birth reflections session with us to debrief our first, traumatic birth. She was my rock all through a pregnancy with lots of stresses, signposted me to a counsellor specialising in birth trauma, and helped us both approach the planned homebirth with positivity and peace. In the end, I had a repeat of pre-eclampsia and needed an emergency caesarean. Lisa brought loving calm into my worst nightmare and her support and that of our second doula Kristal, with the preparation we had done, meant that my son's birth was still the peaceful, positive, healing birth I needed.

Lindsey Middlemiss

Postnatal depression may or may not be linked to birth trauma. Not all birth trauma sufferers will be depressed (some may be, or suffer post-traumatic stress) and certainly not all those suffering will have had an upsetting birth experience, but I do think there is a common thread that not many GPs or therapists acknowledge. I often see women struggling with the transition to motherhood, who are isolated, or unable to reach out for the companionship that is normal for our species. Without a tribe around her, a mother is unable to compare and contrast her parenting style with others, see how other normal babies act, realise that the feelings she is experiencing are shared by other mothers, or pick up tips and information that have benefited others. Without this social support, it is hardly surprising that so many mothers spiral into depression.

The trauma all parents refuse even to think about, the one that sends a cold shudder down any spine, is the loss of a baby. Whether it is miscarriage, abortion or stillbirth, the loss of a child is immense. A family (and their doula) needs love, care and human kindness. More than anything, I think, parents need to be asked what they need, because those needs are so very different for everyone. At first, the shock can be such that knowing what you need can be impossible. It can help to have someone around who can remind you of your options, help you create memories to keep and hopefully prevent regrets or questions later on. Sometimes death comes as a surprise, but sometimes the mother knows she must birth a dead baby. These labours are heartrending but can be beautiful and somehow healing for some mothers. For the doula, it is an enormous honour to be requested to accompany the parents in a birth like this. It makes us humble in the face of the incredible strength that mothers can show.

> *It was without doubt the most mental night of my life, and I felt a massive sense of accomplishment. It wasn't the birth I imagined I'd have, and it was hard to go through it all and not have a baby at the end of it. But no matter what happens with any future pregnancies, I have experienced labour and some form of birth, and I am hugely grateful for that.*
>
> Maisie Hill, after a miscarriage

Michelle Every, a doula who has experienced the loss of a baby herself and who has counselled many mothers and doulas, offers workshops for doulas so that we have the tools to look after ourselves and offer appropriate support to clients dealing with tragedy. She suggests ways to help:

- Choosing to remain present in the moment and engaged in the journey
- Creating a safe space
- Listening
- Acknowledging the loss
- Being honest when they do not know what to say
- Being non-judgemental
- Having no expectations about how the couple will feel
- Being patient, loving and compassionate
- Offering tenderness in touch
- Giving practical, physical and emotional support to the couple, siblings and wider family

- Clearly communicating parents' choices and signposting to longer-term support
- Validating their feelings

Walking this path with clients can be an intensely emotional journey. I will never forget the joy I felt and the tears I shed supporting a mother to birth her baby after a previous loss. Hearing the ecstasy in her voice as she greeted her crying baby was a transcendent experience.

It can be an enormous challenge to support a woman through a labour when everyone knows the baby has died. Yet the birth can still be a positive experience, for all concerned.

Supporting them through the most incredibly beautiful labour was the hardest thing that I had ever done. That beautiful baby never opened her eyes and I prayed so hard that we would be wrong. It has changed the way that I doula, not because it made me fearful of birth, but in part because I rejoice in the miracle of birth. Supporting them made me realise that I really can support anyone. I will carry that baby with me forever.

Mars Lord

The loss of a child seems against nature in our modern world. Despite all the advances in medicine and technology, tragedies still happen. There is nothing we will ever be able to do to prevent them. Sometimes, blame will be sought and found. Sometimes parents will know that Mother Nature just had different plans for that baby. Nothing can ever take away that grief, and nobody should ever try. Loss is a part of a huge percentage of women's lives, yet it is something often suffered in relative silence. Women often carry feelings of shame and guilt with them for the rest of their lives, asking 'What if?' questions of themselves. It is important that parents understand that it is not their fault and, just like with any other birth, they are given choices and treated with kindness and respect and allowed to grieve in the way that feels right for them.

When you are separated from your baby

Usually when parents are separated from their babies, it is because they need a stay in special care. This can be a tumultuous time; getting to know the usually fairly rigid routines of the neonatal intensive care unit can be a rollercoaster of emotions and new challenges. Most units are a lot more parent-friendly now than they once were – it is widely understood that babies do much better with close contact, physical touch and mother's own milk. Research into kangaroo mother care means that continuous skin-to-skin contact with the mother, even for babies who might have been put in incubators, is now more common in units around the country. Babies tucked in against their mother's breasts have their temperature, heart rate and respiration regulated, put on weight more readily and go home more quickly.

Parents need a lot of emotional support during this time. Thankfully there are support structures available, including volunteer peer support from parents who have been through similar experiences. It can be hard, when other families go home with their babies and all your celebrations seem to be on hold. Some parents have no idea if they will ever get to go home with their child at all. Every day can bring a new up or down, as these poorly babies can take turns for the worse or better in the blink of an eye. It can seem that no one knows what to say or how to help with the practicalities of life in NICU. For many parents, once the mother is well enough to be discharged the reality of travelling in from home every day kicks in. The sound of the alarm clock signals another pumping session and life revolves around millilitres, numbers of poos and wees and all the other measurements of how well the baby is doing. Fathers have to go back to work, the dreams of a paternity leave at home with the new baby dashed. The details of home life can be forgotten, and many families will need support even to eat something other than hospital sandwiches.

Your doula will not want you to feel abandoned if this happens to you. On the other hand, she knows how busy and all-consuming NICU life can be and won't want to feel like she's intruding. The contract may say that she was your birth doula and now that relationship is over, but in reality she will want to support you in any way she can. She may have some excellent resources for you; signposts to breastfeeding specialists, for example, or a peer support group, or another client who had a similar experience. She may offer to bring in food, or go shopping for you, or come and help you on the day that you finally bring your baby home. Ask for what you need and if, in the midst of the turmoil, you can't think what you need, see how having a hug and a chat helps – you never know, it might feel good. Likewise, if you need to cut her loose and get on with the job, don't feel guilty – she's a big girl.

We were ready to leave the hospital, all packed up, smiles all around, baby in tow, but everything turned upside-down for us when they found that he had severe jaundice. Just as I had started to get to know our baby, he was taken away, put under powerful lamps in the NICU and fed with a tube. We knew he was in good hands, because the staff were excellent and caring. It took eight days for his levels to settle down. Meanwhile I was busy pumping milk, coming to terms with life and how it had changed. Having our doulas then was a blessing, someone to talk to, a warm hug, and a box of lovely food... just made my day a little better.

Roopsha Sungupta

Multiples

Everything we learn as mothers and doulas is thrown up in the air once there is more than one baby. I've learned on the job, supporting my first twin client when I was a rookie doula. I remember being blown away by the relentlessness of it; the day was one long round of feeding, changing, carrying, cuddling, soothing… and then it started all over again. I would go home exhausted, wondering how she managed to function. I felt useless and worried she thought me useless too. When the twins turned six months and she finally let go of me, I remember her saying that the best thing about me coming around was her little walks round the block by herself. There was always an excuse – a pint of milk, or a letter to post – but those little trips out with just her purse and keys in her pocket – no buggy, no changing bag, no curious people stopping to ask the same old questions, were her sanity-saving moments.

> *At the beginning she helped me persevere with breastfeeding both the boys – something I couldn't be more grateful for now they are nearly six months old, bouncing, happy, and exclusively breastfed the whole way through. She also mopped up a few tears (mine and the twins), took the boys out when I needed to sleep, listened when I wanted to talk about how it was all going and gave the best advice about parenting and motherhood I got from anyone.* Kate Gross[*]

The journey with multiples is a different one from the moment you see more than one tiny beating heart on the ultrasound scan. Mothers can be treated like time bombs, a bundle of risk factors that seem to preclude most of the choices that mothers of singletons have. But just because you are carrying more than one child, doesn't mean you can't

---

[*] Kate Gross tragically died on Christmas Day 2014. Her book *Late Fragments: Everything I want to tell you about this magnificent life* is published by HarperCollins.

keep things as ordinary and normal as medically possible, if that's what you want. People are often surprised that mothers of multiples can have vaginal births and breastfeed. Not all, but many. Just because some mothers need extra help to birth and feed their babies, does that mean we should take the choice away from all of them?

> *With multiples, find out what your hospital trust's [guidelines are] on multiple birth. Decide how you want to birth your babies and don't be "scared" by the fact that there are two not one. You labour once, you push twice but you're already open.* Mars Lord, mother of twins and doula specialising in supporting parents of multiples

A particularly common myth is that a mother will not have enough milk for twins. When asked, I say, 'We only have two boobs because sometimes, we have two babies'. It is genuinely that simple. As milk is made on a supply and demand basis, what you take out will be replaced. In my experience, rather than not enough milk, mothers of twins often have the opposite problem!

Twins clubs can be a supportive way to meet other parents in the same boat and learn some useful tips, but be aware that there may be mothers who genuinely believe that the way they did things is the only way. If you've tried something and it's been a great success, it's tempting to be evangelical, but I've found that parents of multiples generally have as many choices open to them as other parents, and they certainly have the right to find out for themselves what might work, without the complications of myths and other people's personal baggage.

Planning a vaginal birth of twins, or aiming to exclusively breastfeed, or use washable nappies, or bed-share or babywear might present challenges, but all birth and all parenting throws challenges our way. I don't think it's about ditching your dreams, but asking, 'How can I achieve this? What help and support do I need? What information do I need?'

Sometimes just a few words of encouragement and a steer to some useful information can be really supportive. Doulas don't have to be 'your doula' or even know you personally to be a positive presence in a mother's life. This quote left on Selina Wallis's website is a great example:

> I don't know if you remember me complaining on a forum about the pressure for an elective c-section that my doctors were putting me under. Out of the blue you started sending me research around triplet births and any positive birth outcomes you came across. It went on for the rest of the pregnancy and it was wonderful. I was so totally under siege by doctors who were 'national experts' in triplet births, despite only doing an average of three a year! The info you fed me kept me strong and sane.

When I have asked the mums I've worked with who have two or more babies for their advice for other parents of multiples, the answer is always: get help. The workload is that bit more, sleep deprivation can be worse and you may be learning to feed and care for two or three (or more!) very different babies with their own needs, personalities and capabilities.

My clients have used a combination of doula support, friends, family, Homestart, volunteer nanny trainees and mothers' helps to ensure that there is almost always a willing pair of arms. Never underestimate what having help can mean to a mother: I once supported a mum who was raising triplets in a second-floor flat. She couldn't leave home without leaving babies unattended – in the flat while she took the pram downstairs, and while she ran up and down fetching babies. Babies unattended in the lobby scared her witless. It was a major undertaking doing anything at all. A few of us doulas helped her and she didn't pay a penny –

we sought funding to help cover our costs. And when one baby was readmitted to hospital and the mother was ill and couldn't visit, we sat at the baby's bedside texting her regular updates.

Whatever twists or turns your journey takes, your doula might just be the one who manages to say and do just what it is you need. As this mum, Jenny, says:

> What I've realised is that a doula is so much more than someone to support you through labour. Our doula was by my side and shared the entire experience with me, from when I was pregnant, to the birth to the months following. Looking back it feels right to have had a loving, caring, knowledgeable woman share this with me, and I didn't know it back then but I really needed it.
>
> In the early months I found myself experiencing feelings I had never felt before. Despite intense joy at becoming a mother and an all-consuming love for our child I also had moments of feeling incredibly sad and extremely lonely. I didn't feel able to reach out to my friends as I wasn't sure they would understand. One night I was at home upset and the only person I could think of to contact was our doula. I sent her a message admitting my sense of vulnerability, confusion, bewilderment and loneliness. She responded straight away with words of reassurance, love and support. It helped me to make sense of what I was feeling and I am so grateful I was able to reach out to her.

If you have lost a baby, either during pregnancy or after the birth, or are suffering the trauma of shattered dreams of any kind, there are resources that might be useful to you at the end of this chapter. If you need someone to talk to, lift the phone and any doula will be able provide you with some emotional support and point you in the direction of local services.

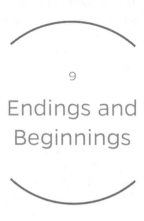

9

Endings and Beginnings

The end of one thing is always the beginning of another. As your baby moves from inside to outside, the birth doula begins to step away to leave your new family to form. I always think of it as like orbits – your doula encircling you still, but at a greater distance as you begin your babymoon. After being on call, sometimes for weeks, and the intensity of the birth, coming home afterwards can be an emotional release for a doula. We all have our rituals, but mine is copious amounts of toast, buckets of builder's tea, a duvet, daytime TV and a nap. I also try to get a massage or an osteopath treatment to nurture my body; birth doula support can take its physical toll! Samantha listens to loud rock music and bakes, Maisie feels a compulsion to have a bath and shave her legs, the need for carb-rich food, sleep and a glass of wine seems pretty universal, and lots of us write our diaries.

When we wake up, we ache to hear how you're getting on, but try not to intrude on this sacred time. When you summon us, we'll come to admire your baby, listen to you recount the story of the birth, fill in any gaps in your memory, and hear how early parenting is playing out for you.

If we have been supporting you through the early weeks, the end of the journey comes in many varied ways. Sometimes we know in advance how much help you'll need and our last, scheduled day arrives so we say our goodbyes. Sometimes, as you get stronger and feel more capable of coping alone, by mutual agreement your doula knocks on the door less and less, until one day you say, 'I don't think I need you any more,' and we know our job is done.

Ongoing relationships (are we friends?)

Some of my closest friends were once clients. Seeing someone express their most basic, primal needs at one of the most vulnerable times in their lives takes all the nice, socially-constructed, smooth edges off a person. If you like what you see then, the likelihood is you like her to the core of her. I often think that if you've seen someone puke and poo and still love them, then it's a friendship for life.

It is a pretty intense adventure we've just been through together. So we could be forgiven for bathing in a warm flush of love for each other. I just saw you do something awesome! You felt how special it is to feel the gentle support and faith of a doula. It can be easy to get carried away on the oxytocin rush. When the music of our dance fades away though, we'll need to stop and take stock. There is a subtle, yet important difference between a doula-client relationship and a friendship of equals. If either side fails to recognise this, it can lead to disappointment and heartbreak.

Doulas aren't 'collectors' of people. Our special role is to support you around the time of childbirth. We can't carry on coming to see you for ever, unless new rules have been mutually agreed. If there comes a time when you no longer need a doula, and I have other mothers who need me, it's time to go, or rewrite our agreement.

So what are the rules? Well, for me, it's about being mindful that the paradigm has changed. I am no longer exclusively the giver and you, the receiver; me the listener, you the sharer. You know very little about my life, my loves, my problems and my worries. If we are to be friends, there will now be times when I can phone you to rant about my crappy day. You, perhaps, can now be my safe haven. When both parties understand that, friendships borne from the doula relationship can be beautiful and fulfilling.

> *Four of my five closest friends were my clients – they were*
> *the first friends I told when I found out I was pregnant,*
> *the ones who I drank margaritas and danced with when*
> *I miscarried. I even stayed with one of them when I was*
> *between homes.* Maisie Hill

Ongoing support

Of course, anyone who thinks that mothers only need support during the childbearing year is away with the fairies. We all need doulaing throughout our parenting lives – I needed a calm voice and some sensible suggestions from a more experienced mother the other day when my adolescent children decided to throw macaroni cheese at each other! I have kept in on-and-off touch with many of my clients as their children grow: when will she sleep through the night? How do I potty train? How do I choose childcare, cope with tantrums, and get her to eat anything green?

I have supported women for as little as two hours and for as long as two years. After a while, the postnatal doula role may morph into something that resembles a cross between a mother's help and a parenting coach or counsellor. Someone to share the practical load of the many mindless tasks of family life, while being genuinely interested in supporting the mum and dad to parent mindfully; creating time and space to consciously reflect on how their parenting journey is developing.

I doulaed a mum back to work. Eased anxiety, supported breastfeeding, reassurance, safety and confidence. Not as 'easy' with a toddler maybe compared to a newborn, but still a valuable source of support for that mum and baby.

Jo Gough

Sometimes, I have been asked back to work with a mother again. This is such an enormous honour. The idea that a woman or couple valued my companionship so much that, despite knowing how it all works and exactly how they'd like things to pan out this time, they still want me around always blows my mind. The dynamic of the relationship is subtly different from the start. That adventure you shared, all that knowledge you have of them, their desires, hopes and dreams, their darkest fears. There is as much talk about the past as about the future. This time, she may worry about having enough love to go around or about getting support for her birth choices. This time, they both know that going with the flow might not be enough of a 'birth plan' to see them through.

Love, love, love repeat clients. No matter how hard I try antenatal appointments just end up chatting and reminiscing! One repeat client has asked me to read at both children's christenings and invited me to every birthday party. I feel like a family member.

Eleanor Fowler

If you've become friends, being asked back wearing your doula hat is an extra honour and so fulfilling for all of you. As one of my client-friends said:

> It made having her as a doula for the birth of my second child even more special, because I love her and love spending time with her, and because I felt even safer and completely at ease with her.

Switching between the roles can be challenging sometimes. Doulaing for close friends or family can present challenges that can take doulas by surprise. We can be much more emotionally invested in the outcome when we doula for friends or family and it can be a little harder to be objective. It can be difficult to stay focused on the task at hand and, from time to time, a doula might need to make it clear where the boundaries lie between doula and friend.

I once realised that I had been acting as an unpaid doula for over a year. I thought I was supporting a friend through a tricky time and I was happy to help. But one day when I had bad news and reached out to her for support, she was unwilling to give it. That relationship was only one-way traffic.

Now, if I realise I am 'falling in friend' with a client, I find myself making an almost childlike declaration. 'Will you be my friend? Someone I can lean on or whinge to sometimes?' I have found this makes it plain how a friendship of equals might have a slightly different flavour to a mother-doula relationship. So far, I've chosen well and those women have easily grasped how the dynamic of our relationship will subtly change once I am no longer their doula.

Debriefing

We talk a lot about debriefing in the doula world. It is shorthand for a whole host of topics and I think it's worth teasing out some of these.

Your doula should never come along to drink your tea and dump her 'stuff' from other births all over you and yours. Not only would that be rather rude, it serves no useful purpose and could prevent you making choices that are right for you. Sadly I sometimes meet women who tell me a doula said something like, 'Ooh, you don't want to do *that*. I had an epidural and it completely ruined my birth and resulted in a forceps delivery and a third degree tear'. That kind of emotionally coercive language is not appropriate.

Even when a doula tries hard not to share those feelings, when she is aware and fully conscious of her baggage, assumptions can still be made. I was reminded of this recently when a woman came to me because she was worried about the blood her baby might be ingesting with her milk because her nipples were cracked and bleeding. She showed me her nipples. Making a face and sucking air in through my teeth, I exclaimed, 'That must be excruciating!'

'Not really', she replied. 'But they are slightly sore'.

She reminded me yet again that we can't just jump in and think we can empathise when we are really just trapped in our own memories and experiences.

Dragging heavy baggage through our doula careers is tough work, so we doula course leaders and mentors try to teach new doulas the habit of debriefing. We can't always help a woman come fully to terms with her experiences of birth and mothering over the short duration of a course, but we can explain why the process is so important, and give her the skills to go forward and find the tools she needs to come to a place of peace, stowing her memories and feelings in a safe place while she supports others.

I don't think we are ever fully debriefed. Our own stories can bite us on the behind, without warning, at any time. As we accompany more women through their birthing and mothering, we can gain a different perspective on our own stories. For many years I thought my first birth was dreadful. I had no positive feelings about it and felt I had been poorly treated and sadly neglected throughout my stay in hospital. As I began to go to births and see the hospital machine in action, I had a slowly-blossoming epiphany: my birth had been wonderful. My midwives had loyally supported me through a long labour, respected my preferences for pain relief, created a private, warm and dimly-lit space for me, encouraged my husband to support me and allowed me to push for well over three hours, which I now know is against their guidelines. I have seen many mothers since have caesareans in almost identical circumstances for 'failure to progress'. Those midwives kept me strong, believed in me and saved me from major surgery.

What coloured my view of the whole story was my experience on the postnatal ward; eleven days of rude, brusque staff, a baby who wouldn't feed and no emotional support until visiting hour arrived. I was bereft and mostly left to myself to try to initiate feeding. It was a lonely, traumatic time. The name of that postnatal ward was reused for a new antenatal ward in the hospital recently; just the sight of the word above the door gave me sweaty palms and a racing heart, fourteen years after my own experiences. Another layer of emotion peeled off. This process can be never-ending. I went and wept, and talked and explored my feelings with a doula friend. After all, no client wants a sweaty ball of adrenaline at her bedside!

Constant reflection on what happened, why it happened, how it made us feel and what we might do differently next time is crucial to the ongoing growth of our doula-selves.

Whether it's reflecting on our own births or those we support, this process is as vital for our well-being as brushing our teeth.

...I don't think that debriefing alone is always enough for every person to not carry their emotional baggage to the births of other women. Reflection is a skill that must be learnt and it requires constant refinement...To me, not allowing myself to impact on births and birth choices is actually practising a kind of mindfulness.

Kath Harbisher

Part of making friends with our own stories is about understanding where we have come from. And when we understand that, we can make a little more sense of where we're going. When doulas 'get' it, it comes naturally to support their clients through this process. Stories are our life-blood. Listening to the stories of my mentor and friend Linda Quinn, who has been a doula for over forty years, has taught me far more than any book.

Doulas hear a lot of stories. I think we should listen to them hard, treat them with reverence and support a mother until she can honour her story, own it, and hopefully, feel pride in it. We listen and realise that sometimes mothers need more ears than just ours. Sometimes mothers need to talk to a professional of some kind. Sometimes it's the partner who needs to speak and be heard. Bystanders and companions have a story to share and emotion to make sense of too.

Some people call us 'birth keepers'. I think we could also be called 'story keepers'. Doulas celebrate a rich, female oral tradition that goes back to the dawn of time. Storytelling is our hearth, our health and our teacher.

Everything that happens and every word spoken around a mother during the childbearing year stays with her. The story is told and retold. She rolls the narrative around in her head for years after. If that story is painful, the threads of the tale may entangle her. But positive stories weave wonderful webs and create insight, self-awareness and growth.

> I realise that pain, whether physical or emotional, passes. That's what you taught me when giving birth to J. You said it'll pass, let it pass, and that felt so relevant at the time, and I apply that now when it comes to sticky situations. I've got you to thank for that. If anything's going to register, it's sure to register when giving birth, and it did.
>
> Nikki

We constantly tell stories. Ever mindful of confidentiality, we weave our tales in safe circles and protect the identities of the central characters. Our very system of mentoring is based on this sharing of the tale. In the sharing, it takes on a life of its own: as mentor helps mentee to reflect, understand, see from a different angle, the narrative can shape-shift and reveal new meanings, new teachings, new epiphanies.

Feeding back

After you have walked the path with your doula, and once you feel ready to continue the journey without her, it will be time to part. Your doula will have learned so much from you. If she is a mentored doula, she will ask you for some formal feedback, which will be sent directly to her mentor. She should have made you aware of this system from the outset, so that you took her on happy to know that your story will be shared with one other doula, who will receive your feedback and use it to help the mentored doula learn and grow.

As mentors we are constantly humbled by the feedback that we receive from parents about their doula. At a time when life is very full and extremely tiring, the very fact that a mother would put pen to paper is amazing. The gushing comments that show so clearly how much that doula support was appreciated are wonderful. The constructive criticism is even more appreciated, because it helps us all reflect on how we can improve, perhaps becoming more understanding or sensitive, or flexible, or organised in the process.

I think a fascination and a reverence for feedback, debriefing and the power of stories is one of the defining characteristics of doula mentors. Watching and helping a doula to blossom, as an individual as well as a doula, is also a large part of why we are drawn to the role. As Michelle Every, doula mentor coordinator, says, the pleasure comes from

> ...see[ing] a new doula discover their potential and hav[ing] the confidence to run with it.

If your doula is a recognised doula, she hopes you will give her feedback too. Sometimes doulas ask for formal feedback. Mostly we look forward to that last visit when we chat about how things have gone, how you're feeling about the whole experience and listen carefully for things we could have done better. Sometimes we are bowled over by thank-you cards and presents. These are never expected, but treasured forever.

Sometimes, rarely we hope, things don't work out as beautifully as everyone hoped. I think it is right and proper to include some words about when having a doula isn't everything it was cracked up to be. There are all sorts of reasons why this might happen. Usually either the parents or the doula, or both, ignored early signs that their personalities might clash. Sometimes, neither party communicated as effectively with the other as they could have. Sometimes, very sadly, a doula hasn't fully debriefed her own experiences, or is a bit evangelical about what she believes birth 'should' be. Sometimes we forget to validate our client's feelings. Perhaps an off-the-cuff remark on a bad or tired day really rankles with our clients. Sometimes we jump to conclusions and make assumptions. If these things happen during pregnancy or after the baby is born, it can be upsetting, but if it's during labour, mothers can feel traumatised by the promise of unconditional support that wasn't forthcoming.

> I wanted comforting, but I felt that she was distant, silent. I kept telling her I was scared, she kept telling me to switch my mind off, stop worrying. But I had been pushing for several hours with still no sign of baby. People talk about instinctual birth; all my instincts told me that baby was stuck, but she didn't hear me. To cut a long story short, I felt totally abandoned.

Often it is things that could seem insignificant that mean so much to mothers. It can feel lonely if everyone in the room is watching a head emerge from your vagina and no one is looking at you. It can seem intrusive if a doula contacts you too much. Or you can feel ignored if she doesn't get in touch enough. Perhaps she doesn't really understand what you need. Perhaps she's missed the fear or private pain you're desperately trying to share. It is the doula's responsibility to try her best to build a relationship of trust and openness. But communication is a two-way street, so if you're not entirely happy, talk about it with your doula. Her job is not to get defensive, but to really listen to you and work out whether she can be the doula you need. If she can't, she may find you someone who can.

Having a doula should result in you feeling like you are being

given space, confidence and empowerment.

Boo Newns

If you're not feeling that way, something needs to change. Hopefully, all that will be needed is a conversation to take your relationship onto a deeper, more even footing.

But when a relationship breaks down completely, especially at a time in your life when you are feeling extra-vulnerable, it's good to know that there is support out there. If you approach Doula UK, our organisation will do everything in its power to hear you and find you the appropriate support. One very good reason for a group of autonomous, self-employed individuals to band together to form an organisation is to provide the public with checks and balances, a Code of Conduct and other guidance documents, a complaints procedure and a general level of accountability for our actions.

Thankfully, complaints are rare. The vast majority of doula-client relationships are fulfilling for all concerned – to the extent that I speak to many parents who say that no amount of money would be enough to adequately repay what they feel they have received from their doula. Sometimes I get asked by parents what they can do to show their appreciation. I always tell parents to look at the doula's website to see if she has made her preferences clear. One doula I know states clearly not to give her flowers; not just because she is allergic, but because she feels the money could be better spent elsewhere. I tend to agree with her; I am up-front with clients that a tip will go down much better with me. Over-payments from parents who can afford it make it financially viable for me to support parents who are less well-off. Being a doula is a hand-to-mouth occupation for most of us, so extras and treats for the family are often in short supply. I am currently feeling all loved-up and grateful to a couple who have given my family a few nights away in a beautiful holiday home. For a family that rarely gets holidays, it couldn't have been a better gift; given and received with love.

But I'll tell you what lights my fire more than any gift for myself, and that's 'paying it forward'. For anyone not familiar with this phrase, it means passing on what you have received. So if you have felt heard, understood, approved of, supported, informed or just helped with some of the practical tasks of parenthood, pass on some of that support. Be that friend with a non-judgemental smile, cook that new family a meal, pass on those old baby clothes to someone who needs them. It certainly does take a village to raise a child, but what we forget in that old cliché is that it takes all of us to create strong, capable, happy and healthy mothers, too.

So many of us doulas become doulas and mentors precisely because of the support we received when we were starting out. Paying it forward is an idea rooted at the heart of all we do.

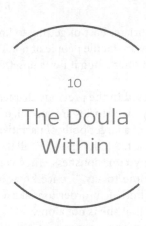

10

The Doula Within

Leaning in to listen

I believe doulas should never forget that we have two eyes, two ears and one mouth. We watch and we listen twice as much as we speak. We know that the words tumbling out of a mother's mouth are necessary, cathartic and are often helping her make sense of a confusing situation or clearing the way for a different way of looking at things.

I try to show a mother that I approve of her and whatever she has to say. I try to do this with my body language, my focus on her and by helping to make her comfortable. We English doulas often do this by offering and sharing cups of tea. Hugging a mug, hiding behind it, taking a sip, setting it down – all these things take away a little self-consciousness, punctuate the conversation and allow a little rumination before responding.

Sometimes touch – hugs, a hand on a shoulder or holding a hand – can be just what a woman needs. Other times, it doesn't feel appropriate. Part of getting to know my clients is working out if they are tactile people or not. Personally, I'd feel bereft if you didn't offer a hug if I was upset. You might be the direct opposite.

I also, as discussed in the previous chapter, try to put away my own 'stuff'. My own stories are special, of course, but they have become part of a larger body of narratives floating round in my head and heart. All those stories, all those women; their voices populate my consciousness. They come to mind as I listen and inspire me to say, 'I once knew a woman who...' or 'Some women find...' in order to make a suggestion or to show this mother that she is not alone.

I work with so many women who tell me that, on top of the worries and concerns they have, they feel guilty, silly or bothersome to feel that way. I find myself saying, 'It's OK to feel this way, it's entirely understandable you feel this way, many, many mothers feel like this. In fact, it's hardly surprising you feel this way!'

Sometimes, women need to have their emotion named. The feelings can be tumultuous, shapeless and undefined. A timely suggestion that it sounds like she's feeling angry, resentful or any number of adjectives or even that it must be hard, dealing with all of this, can help. Defining, naming and labelling are ways that human beings cope, control and eventually conquer chaos – be that physical or emotional.

All doulas can relate to the story of the woman who talks. And talks. And talks. And we listen. We nod our heads. We smile, we frown at the appropriate moments. We interject with the right noises at the right points. We might ask a few open questions. After quite some time, she will say something like, 'I think I might...' or, 'I could...'. We say: 'That sounds like a brilliant idea!' She gathers herself, looks more settled and at home in her body and says, 'Thanks for that advice, it really helped!'

We so often have the answers inside us. Sometimes we might need information, people or answers to specific questions as pieces of the jigsaw puzzle – and a doula can help with that. But at the end of the day, only the parents know the right answer.

Doulas are born, not made

Becoming a doula is about so much more than understanding the ins and outs of pregnancy, birth and beyond. Our journey is as much about getting to know ourselves; our strengths, our weaknesses, our judgement buttons. It's about exploring and reflecting constantly on our boundaries; knowing where the doula role begins and ends is crucial. It's about nurturing the doula inside ourselves, so she blossoms. We are also encouraged to think about how to walk the high wire of work-life balance. But most of all, it is about coming to terms with the fact that doula is not what you do, it is who you are.

As well as the families I support, I have loved and still get intense pleasure from supporting other women on their doula journeys. The few days we spend together on their doula preparation course is often the first time that some women have spent time nurturing themselves. It is sometimes the first time they have experienced a women's circle. We reflect a lot on community and the gaping chasm it leaves in our lives when it is missing. We also reflect on our own paths as women and mothers and begin to make sense of our story so far. It is a time to stop and look back along the path we have come before exploring the way ahead. It is a time to connect with like-minded women and be reminded what strong, creative, brave women we really are.

What form doula education takes and what it should encompass has been a hot topic over the years. If doulas are not medical, if we're not actually doing anything clinical, what exactly are we teaching doulas? Here in the UK, we course providers work closely together and with Doula UK to make sure that what we are offering gives women the best possible preparation for supporting families with that three-legged doula-stool of practical help, emotional support and information. We work to a core curriculum and regularly reflect on the responsibilities that go with being a doula course leader.

Once the course is over, the opportunity to reflect, learn and grow continues. Working with a mentor means new doulas have companionship, guidance and wise counsel. Her mentor is her doula; providing unconditional, non-judgemental support and friendship. If you are a parent thinking of working with a doula, don't rule out the possibility of having a mentored doula. They are not only typically cheaper than a recognised doula, but you are also tapping into the experience of her mentor. So it's kind of like two doulas for the price of one.

Being mentored or, as we put it within Doula UK, the 'recognition process', isn't easily defined. A doula will work through a number of journeys with clients and debrief them with her mentor. So if you ask a mentored doula to support you, she will explain that the circle of confidentiality will include her mentor. You'll be asked to send a feedback form to the mentor after your journey together is over. The real learning – about what it means to be a doula, how to effectively support families and what in ourselves helps and hinders our doulaing – necessarily begins after our doula course is finished. Parents and babies are our best teachers.

However, there will come a time when the mentor 'recognises' that the new doula has developed into a reflective, sensitive, empathic supporter and will carry the name doula with reverence and pride. The doula meets with her mentor and, usually over tea and cake, they look back over the journey they have travelled together and the mentored doula is reborn as a recognised doula.

In the last decade I have seen the world change from one in which I was mistaken for a 'dealer' or a 'jeweller' to one in which many have a vague understanding of the term doula. We work much more closely with our midwifery colleagues and are building strong links with other organisations working to support women during the childbearing year. But bearing the name 'doula' is still a funny old business; there are some who are suspicious or dismissive. A few are downright hostile. It can be dispiriting sometimes to encounter attitudes from those who don't understand. We women who serve need dignity, a thick skin, passion and commitment. There are many of us who don't even earn enough to pay tax and most of us could be earning more doing something else. Many of us do something else *as well* in order to feed our families.

We are dragged out of bed at 3am, leave our families, sometimes for days on end, and bore everyone stupid talking about labour hormones, skin-to-skin contact and nipples at the dinner table. Doulas are born, not made; it goes to the heart of us. So we can sometimes be difficult to live with. This vocation necessarily has an effect on those around us. Our partners and children, in particular, bear the brunt.

Debbie's husband says:

> I hate worrying about you when you're at a birth, especially long ones when you're not eating properly and driving home in the early hours tired. The good is seeing the secret frustrated dream become a true life passion and the inner glow you have supporting these women on their journey.

Despite the interruptions to family life, the nights without sleep and the clothes stained with various bodily fluids, this work is addictive. Watching women become mothers and men become fathers is, quite literally, the biggest privilege we can imagine.

I once left a cosy little cottage after a long night's home birth support. I was toasty warm after hours of running up and down to the kitchen to boil kettles to keep the birth pool water the right temperature. My soul was glowing with the knowledge that she had achieved her home birth despite a long list of challenges. As I walked to the bus stop, the snow crunched under foot. It was so early, mine were the only footprints. The city was almost silent. Above me, the sky was a deep, cloudless blue, streaked with the orangey tint of sunrise. It felt like the world had been cleaned, remade, reborn.

I had damp socks, meconium on my T-shirt and blood on my trousers. I had not slept in 36 hours, and had eaten a handful of peanuts and a chocolate biscuit in the last twelve. But I couldn't wipe the grin off my face. I felt like shouting at the top of my voice: 'Don't you realise, a *child* was just born in that house? A mother was stronger than she ever thought possible. A father was her rock. She *did* it, against all the odds. Why aren't you worshipping her?'

The biggest gift being a doula has given me is a renewed love and respect for women. Both the mothers I support and my sister doulas have taught me that women need women. A doula friend, Ellie Cook, says that doulaing has been:

A chance to connect with women on a completely honest and intimate level. Something I denied myself for a long time through fear. But something I always desperately needed. I hadn't had any real female friends since I was in secondary school. It's like coming home again.

My biggest lesson has been that there is always more to know. Every story I witness play out, every parent I get to know, reminds me how much I still have to learn. I hope anyone reading this book will bear in mind that these short chapters of thoughts and observations, together with the voices of some generous contributors, aim to begin to explain why doulas matter by showing you something of what doula support, in all its complexity, can look like. If you are thinking of booking a doula, take everything I have said as a starting point; do your own research, listen to your own heart. You will know if it's right for you.

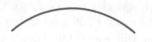

Further Reading and Resources

Books

Barnes, B., Badley, S.G. *Planning for a healthy baby*, Ebury, 1990.

Buckley, S. *Gentle Birth, Gentle Mothering: A Doctor's Guide to Natural Childbirth and Gentle Early Parenting Choices*, Celestial Arts, 2009.

England, P. and Horowitz, R. *Birthing From Within*, Alburquerque, New Mexico: Partera Press, 1998.

Evans, K. Bump. *How to make, Grow and Birth a Baby*, Myriad Editions, 2014.

Evans, K. *The Food of Love: Your Formula for Successful Breastfeeding*, Myriad Editions, 2008.

Gaskin, I.M. *Ina May's Guide to Childbirth*, Vermillion, 2008.

Gerhardt, S. *Why Love Matters*, Routledge, 2004.

Hazard, L. *The Father's Homebirth Handbook*, Pinter & Martin, 2008.

Kemeny, N. *Nurturing New Families*, Pinter & Martin, 2014.

La Leche League International, *Sweet Sleep*, Pinter & Martin, 2014.

La Leche League International, *The Womanly Art of Breastfeeding*, Pinter & Martin, 2010.

Marshall, H., Klaus, M.H., Kennel, J.H. and Klaus, P.H. *The Doula Book*, Da Capo Lifelong Books; 3rd revised edition, 2012.

Palmer, G. *The Politics of Breastfeeding – When Breasts are Bad for Business*, Pinter & Martin, 2009.

Simkin, P. *The Birth Partner: A Complete Guide to Childbirth for Dads, Doulas, and Other Labor Companions*, 4th revised edition, Harvard Common Press, 2013.

Stockton, A. *Gentle Birth Companions: doulas serving humanity*, McCubbington Press, 2010.

Stockton, A. *Birth Space, Safe Place: Emotional Well-Being Through Pregnancy and Birth*, Findhorn Press, 2009.

Stadlen, N. *What Mothers Do – Especially When It Looks Like Nothing*, Piatkus, 2005.

Stadlen, N. *How Mothers Love*, Piatkus, 2011.

Sundin, J. *Birth skills: Proven pain-management techniques for your labour and birth*, Vermillion, 2008.

Taylor, E. *Becoming Us: 8 Steps to Grow a Family that Thrives*, Three Turtles Press, 2014.

Websites

Doula UK articles on what a doula is and what we do
doula.org.uk/content/what-doula
doula.org.uk/content/what-do-doulas-do

The origins of the doula – a global perspective
adelastockton.co.uk

A round up on the research on doula support
evidencebasedbirth.com/the-evidence-for-doulas

Pre-conception and conception information and support
foresight-preconception.org.uk

Finding a doula in your area
doula.org.uk/find-a-doula

Honouring the last days of pregnancy
mothering.com/articles/the-last-days-of-pregnancya-place-of-
in-between

Evidence around induction of labour
sarawickham.com/tag/induction

Maternity and human rights
birthrights.org.uk
humanrightsinchildbirth.com
rosesrevolution.com
aims.org.uk

Positive peer support
positivebirthmovement.org
tellmeagoodbirthstory.com

Childbirth preparation
ahaparenting.com
bellybelly.com.au/birth/birth-plan-can-you-planbirth

Comfort and control during childbirth
birthunplugged.blogspot.co.uk/2010/11/traditional-
birthsecrets-rebozo.html
natalhypnotherapy.co.uk
thewisehippo.com
thehypnobirthingcentre.co.uk
activebirthcentre.com
birthlight.co.uk
nct.org.uk/courses/antenatal/antenatal-services/relax-stretch-
and-breathe-nct-yoga-pregnancy

Inspiration, information and choice
aims.org.uk AIMS booklets, especially Am I allowed
which.co.uk/birth-choice

anthrodoula.blogspot.co.uk/2011/06/informed-choiceand-brain-acronym.html

pregnancy.com.au/birth-choices/homebirth/ out-of-the-laboratory-back-to-the-darkened-room.shtml

sarahbuckley.com/articles

Second stage of labour and the immediate postnatal period
wombecology.com/?pg=fetusejection
thebirthpause.com
bellybelly.com.au/baby/why-its-best-to-avoid-putting-a-hat-on-your-newborn-baby/

Third stage of labour – birthing your placenta
midwifethinking.com/2010/08/26/the-placenta-essentialresuscitation-equipment
kangaroomothercare.com
sarahbuckley.com/leaving-well-alone-a-naturalapproach-to-the-third-stage-of-labour
aims.org.uk/pubs3.htm
placentanetwork.com/research-and-articles/placenta-the-forgotten-chakra-by-robin-lim/

The science of infant sleep
isisonline.org.uk
babymanualnotincluded.com

Postnatal support
thebirthhub.co.uk/closing-bones/
bellybelly.com.au/post-natal/birth-releaseceremony-healing-when-your-birth-didnt-go-to-plan
oneplusone.org.uk/content_topic/becoming-aparent/common-problems-for-new-parents

Feeding – issues, politics and advocacy
The WHO Code who.int/nutrition/publications/code_english. pdf
analyticalarmadillo.co.uk

Unbiased information on breastmilk substitutes
firststepsnutrition.org/newpages/infants/infant_ feeding_
    infant_milks_UK.html
babymilkaction.org

Feeding support
kellymom.com
abm.me.uk
breastfeedingnetwork.org.uk
laleche.org.uk
nct.org.uk/parenting/feeding

The science and psychology of parenting
normalfed.com/onion *Onion Mothers and Shoe Salesmen*
www.analyticalarmadillo.co.uk/2012/01/message-for-
    expectantnew-parents.html

Fathers/Partners
daddynatal.co.uk
birthingawareness.com/birthing-for-blokes
fatherstobe.org
fatherhoodinstitute.org

Unassisted birth
aims.org.uk/Journal/Vol19No3/itIsIllegal.htm
birthrights.org.uk/library/factsheets/UnassistedBirth.pdf
unassistedchildbirth.com

Special care
parenting.com/article/leaving-baby-behind

Birth trauma and mental health support
birthtraumaassociation.org.uk
pandasfoundation.org.uk
petalscharity.org

Losing a child
uk-sands.org

Debriefing
birchtreebeginnings.co.uk/birth-debriefing

Becoming a doula
doula.org.uk/content/journey-being-doula
doula.org.uk/content/becoming-doula

Doula UK approved training courses
doula.org.uk/content/list-doula-uk-recognised-courses

Unashamed plug for Maddie's course and websites
developingdoulas.co.uk
thebirthhub.co.uk
maddiemcmahon.com

Michel Odent doula course
paramanadoula.com

Living with a doula and doulas reflect on their role
wonderfullymadebelliesandbabies.blogspot.co.uk/2014/03/
    my-wifes-doula.html
anthrodoula.blogspot.co.uk/2011/09/being-doula-is-hard
jodithedoula.com/2013/03/02/no-free-births
northeastdoulas.com/blog/becoming-doulashusband

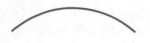

Acknowledgments

Rather too many cups of tea and chocolate biscuits were consumed while gestating this book. A small, black and white kitten reminded me that babies need attention and laptop wires are nice to chew. Any typos, I blame on her.

Chris, my husband, grammar fiend and plain speaker, gave me the highest praise possible: he didn't rewrite whole swathes of the text. For that, and his never-ending belief that I could do it, I am grateful.

Daniel and Libby, my children – well, thanks for putting up with me.

To the whole community of doulas, near and far: you gave me your voices, your strength, your faith, your wisdom, endless inspiration and, on occasion, a room of my own and a shoulder to cry on. You are all loved. Special thanks to Sophie Messager for her help with the resources at the end of the book, Mars Lord, Lindsey Middlemiss, Vicki Williams, Bridget Baker and Adela Stockton.

My doula-mother, Linda Quinn: you could never teach me all you know in a lifetime. Thank you for nurturing me so lovingly through so many doula transitions.

All the mothers and fathers and babies I have supported: thank you – your stories populate my soul and have taught me to be humble. Those who honoured me with their stories for this book deserve special mention too. I hope I have cradled your words with the reverence they deserve.

Special mention to Susan Last, my editor. You truly have doulaed me through the birth of this book. Thank you for your love and wisdom.

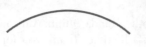

Index

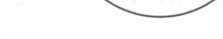